The Gurus' Guide to Reflexology

CU00920806

Contributions from:

Arve Fahlvik – Balancing Hormones

Katie Gunn – Baby Reflex

Susan Quayle – Puberty – a Child's Journey to Sexual Maturity

AOR – Maternity Reflexology – The Basics to Treating Safely

Heidi Armstrong – Chinese Medicine and Pregnancy Reflexology

Dorothy Kelly – My Approach to Fertility Reflexology,
with Naturopathic Support

Sally Earlam – Therapeutic Relationships during Maternity

Heinrike Bergmans – Reflexology as a Communication Tool between
the Mother and her Unborn Baby

Jenni Tribe – Quantum Physics and the Incoming Soul

Jane Sheehan (Norwich) – Menopause

Section for Support for Reflexologists and their clients:

Maura O'Shea – Top 5 Tips for Successful Breastfeeding

Teri Woods – Lifestyle Choices for a Healthy Mind and
Body during Menopause

Beverley Higham – Aromatherapy and Reflexology for the Menopause

Amanda Thomas – Traditional Acupuncture and how it Benefits Fertility

It is by no means a complete guide and we aim to cover the theme of
Cancer in the next book in this series – *Book 3*.

The Gurus' Guide to Reflexology

Hormones: Puberty, Fertility, Pregnancy, Maternity, Menopause

Edited by Jane Sheehan

www.footreading.com
www.lecturedespieds.fr
www.letturadeipiedi.it

"The Gurus' Guide to Reflexology – Book 2" by Jane Sheehan
First Edition 2020

Published by
Jane Sheehan
Weighbridge House
Southport Road
Scarisbrick
Nr Ormskirk
Lancs
L40 8HQ
England
www.footreading.com

ISBN 978-0-9571071-6-8

Design by Nicki Averill Design

Contents

5: Maternity Reflexology – The Basics to Treating Safely

Support for Reflexologists and their Clients

Introduction
by Jane Sheehan HMAR

Introduction
by Jane Sheehan
HMAR

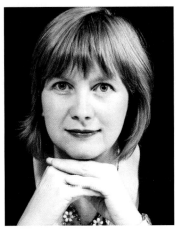

This is the second book in the **"Gurus' Guide to Reflexology"** Series. Book one was about reflexology in general. This book is themed on puberty, menstruation, (in)fertility, pregnancy, maternity and menopause.

Our aim in writing this book is to bring some of the best gurus together in one place to share their knowledge and to whet your appetite to learn more. Whether you are a new reflexologist or have been practicing for years, we think you will find something in this book to inspire you.

I must admit that when I first mooted this book, I was interested in producing a book to help my fellow reflexologists when they had requested this topic. However, once I started pulling together all the chapters and speaking to the various gurus, I became fascinated. In setting out to help others, I have ended up learning heaps myself.

My first introduction to all things "hormones" came about when I met Suzanne Enzer at her talk in London. Suzanne was pretty much famous in reflexology circles for her "Hat talk". She explained the different stages of life and the effects that hormones had on those stage by placing a series of props into a straw hat on her head. She would talk about the birds and the bees, and hey presto, she would produce a bird and a bee on a stick and poke them into her hat. You never knew what she would produce next! What it looked like at the end of the talk, well, imagine a milliner's worst nightmare! It was certainly memorable.

Suzanne also taught me about "Coffee/Cola legs". She said that a reflexologist called Val Groom in Essex had studied what her clients ate and drank and noticed that sometimes a client with undiagnosed infertility (where they had had all the tests but their consultant could find no reason for their inability to fall pregnant) would have what she called "Coffee/Cola legs". She said to look for a spongy feeling behind the malleolus. She told us to measure the circumference around this area of the leg then ban the client from having any caffeinated drinks – no coffee, tea, hot chocolate, cola etc. Then a week later to measure the circumference again. The dimensions would be greatly reduced, and the sponginess would be gone. She reported improved results in clients falling pregnant after this.

I had such a client. I too banned her from caffeinated drinks. The client reported back that her husband said, "Whatever you are doing, keep doing it" and that her moods were less stormy and calmer. She fell pregnant. When it got to Christmas, she visited her family who had purchased enough diet coke for her visit. She no longer drank it because of my instructions. She was utterly horrified at the amount of diet coke stacked up awaiting her. I asked how many she used to drink. "A case a day" she replied.

It was many years later that I read an article in the Daily Mail about a study to show how caffeine impairs the healthy functioning of the fallopian tube by impairing the contractions of the walls of the fallopian tube which are needed to carry the eggs to the womb. **(https://www.dailymail.co.uk/health/article-1390105/Why-cups-coffee-day-hinder-conception-25-cent.html)**

To my knowledge, I have never met Val Groom, but I know that because of her, via Suzanne Enzer, I was able to help my client.

I am hoping that by producing and editing this book, I will be helping you to help your clients too.

We plan to bring out the third book in this series on the theme of Cancer.

Jane Sheehan

Balancing Hormones, the Other Way

by Arve Fahlvik

Balancing Hormones, the Other Way
by Arve Fahlvik

To balance hormones is something everyone needs. Whatever life situation you are in or eventually what diseases you have, it is very likely that your hormonal system is overloaded and out of balance. This is why I almost always start on this process on new clients, even if they come to get help with something that is not related to hormones. For example, elbow pain. There is usually something behind the surface. This text will describe a way of doing this that is not common among foot reflexologists, and it will only be about the glands located in the head.

On the majority of reflexology charts you will find the head projected on the big toe. And the head is where you find the primary glands to regulate the hormonal systems of the body. First, forget about the big toe. The head is projected on all toes. All properties of the body are best treated when it is done on the right projection. There are no "one size fits all" projections that can be the best one for all issues. Clinical experience shows that the best toes to treat any kind of mental stress are the fourth and the fifth. Even though they are smaller than the big toe, they are the best indicators for high activity level in the neural and hormonal system of the head.

The smaller size (of the toes) can obviously provide less detail. This leads to the next thing you can forget, the details of the glands on your charts. All you need to know is that the head is projected on the outermost segment of these toes. All sore spots on those toes are indicating some kind of mental stress. Just trust the signals from the body and treat these spots. Relieve these spots by massaging them, then your client will improve somehow.

Sometimes, you will not need to think more about that elbow pain. This treatment starts a process where the client will have spare resources to focus on the major things in life. The elbow problem might disappear by itself when the person as a whole heals. When the hormones are in balance the body has spare resources to take care of such details as a painful elbow by itself.

The practice

The small size of these toes makes it inconvenient to only work with your hands. A small stick gives you good access to all the interesting areas and strains your hands less. There are four separate areas on the projection of the head that one can "identify" and treat. It is not so that you should ignore what is outside these areas. They are just a guide for beginners for where to look first and indicate where most tension is to be found. By the way, toes? I actually prefer to start most of my treatments on the hands, so for the hormones it will be on the fingers. The body does not express the exact same stress on the fingers as on the toes. There will be some overlap, but best results are achieved if both fingers and toes are treated. For convenience, the following pictures only show fingers, but it will be exactly the same on the toes.

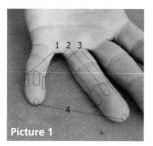

Picture 1

Picture 1 indicates the reflexes. Tension in area 2 shows some correlation to sleep issues, menstruation cycles and heart rhythm. Area 4 shows some correlation to sensory/motor issues.

It can be a good idea to roll the stick on the toe at first. This is to locate the most interesting areas, and to not suddenly inflict pain.

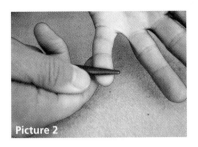
Picture 2

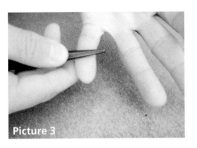
Picture 3

As the treatment goes on, these tender areas will be reduced, and you will need the tip of the stick to access them. You might also have to go deeper to reach them. Picture 4 indicates the location where you can go deep. When you slide between the positions indicated in picture 4 and 5 you might find a structure that feels like a string. Lots of work is needed there.

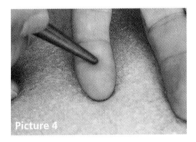
Picture 4

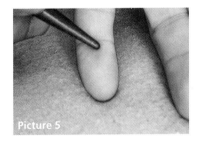
Picture 5

On some clients the toes are most painful, on other clients the fingers. Check the client to figure out where to focus. Usually I spend 4 to 5 minutes on each toe. Sometimes twice as much can be needed. In some cases, I treat for 10 or 14 days consecutively, and sometimes for even more than two hours. Use some lubrication to protect the skin. Sometimes, especially in the beginning, the tissue can make a sound when you treat with a stick. During the progress of the treatment the sound will change, and eventually disappear. When you have some experience with this way of treating you will be able to feel the difference in the tissue representing older and newer tension.

I use this treatment in a variety of situations with good results. Just to mention a few: sleeping issues, AD/HD, Tourettes, cancer, general stress, fibromyalgia, allergies and anxiety.

The bonus

I like to involve the clients in the treatment process. If they come to be fixed without any involvement, they'd better go to a doctor. Here is one way of involving them.

The brain is also projected on the tongue, and the glands are located on the midline. Sometimes a furrow can be seen there. This furrow can indicate more than hormonal issue, but that is outside the scope of this text. I encourage them to use their toothbrush on the tongue, and mostly on the midline. Picture 6 should clearly indicate where the brushing is needed.

About the author

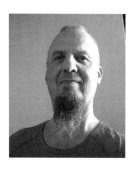

Arve Fahlvik started with Reflexology in 1997. Teacher of Karl Axel Lind method of reflexology, full body reflexology, since 2005. Board member of International Council of Reflexologists since 2017, with responsibility for the research committee. Vice chair of RiEN from May 2011 to May 2013. Board member of Norske Naturterapeuters Hovedorganisasjon (NNH) from May 2005 to May 2009. Leader of group for full body reflexology in NNH from its start in 2005 until 2016. Initiator of the Definition Reflexology and the related International Reflexology Teachers Conference projects.

You can learn more from **https://arvefahlvik.wordpress.com/** Or email him at **arve@fahlvik.org**

Baby Reflex

by Katie Gunn

Baby Reflex
by Katie Gunn

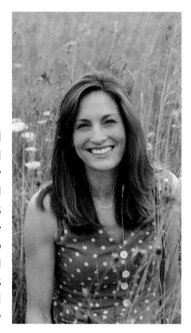

Having trained in the Baby and Toddler Reflex techniques before I (Katie Gunn) took over from Jenny in 2017 (after her retirement), I knew how effective the routines were and the difference they were making not only to babies but also parents and guardians as well. I chose to learn these techniques because of my own personal experience after the birth of my first child.

We live in a world now where we are made to feel that in order to be a 'good' parent, we must look to an 'expert', we are bombarded with books, usually all saying differing things. As a parent it becomes confusing and as a first time parent we cling to these books, hoping they will help to guide us through…but in doing so, many of us lose the ability to trust our gut instinct and follow the cues that our babies give us.

I feel very passionate about teaching parents and giving them not only a skill for life, but also a tool that they can use any time & anywhere to help reconnect and bond with their child. I believe we have a generation of parents that are struggling to connect with their babies. We live in a world that is so busy, noisy and all consuming. With the rise of social media there never seems to be a time for silence, time to observe and time to grow.

I was one of those parents. After the birth of my first child, I looked to a book to help me 'take back some control', I laugh out loud when I think about this phrase now. When I look back, I feel angry that those first five months of my baby's life were lost to me. After months of trying and 'failing' to follow the routine, the book was finally binned! It was only then that I realised I'd completely lost the ability to follow my instinct and I was unable to read any of the cues my little one was giving me. I felt sad and angry. But I knew I could recover all that was lost through the power of touch. And that is how my journey of working with little people using reflexology began. I felt calmer, relaxed and more in 'control' than ever before.

With Baby Reflex we not only teach parents the techniques but also empower them to listen to their gut, be patient and look to follow the cues that their baby gives them. It is very much a collaboration between parent and child, with boundaries being set on both sides. A focus on mum's own health and wellbeing is also an important part of our discussions. Research has shown that if mum is relaxed and calm, she is much more likely to be able to regulate the needs of her baby. Supporting her child's emotional and physical wellbeing is without doubt a catalyst for enabling her baby to flourish. We also know that the first 4 years of a child's life are effectively its blueprint. By establishing regular, loving and positive touch, especially in those first four years, we are helping to build future stable foundations for our child's mental, emotional and physical wellbeing. I believe these classes are more important than ever before. Helping to support parents on their journey is a privilege and I'm forever thankful that I'm able to be part of their tribe. As the saying goes, it takes a village to raise a child.

Jenny Lee, MCSP MAR, the founder of Baby Reflex is both a Chartered Physiotherapist and a Qualified Reflexologist who has been working with mothers and young children for many years. Jenny has also carried out several pilot research studies in conjunction with those children's GPs, which were designed to examine the effects of Reflexology treatments on asthmatic children.

The results of those studies revealed numerous benefits for those children, for example, reduced asthma; better sleep patterns; greater ability to relax; a much improved "quality of life ", and perhaps, most important of all, an enjoyment by those children of the actual treatment of reflexology.

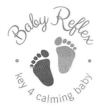

Having been asked for more information by mothers who had seen the effect of Reflexology, Jenny decided to introduce this new and exciting concept as an easily learned and effective therapy called **"Baby Reflex"**.

Baby Reflex is a series of specially adapted reflexology techniques originally developed for increasing that all important bonding between parents and babies. Further development of the techniques has enabled parents to also help to ease and relieve many normal baby discomforts in their own child.

Baby Reflex has proved to be very popular with both parents and young children and is safe to use with babies aged 4 weeks and onwards.

Most parents have either tried, or heard of, the many benefits of reflexology. With the modern climate of parents seeking alternative health treatments, Baby Reflex offers parents the benefits of a safe, non-invasive, drug free and natural therapy that they can apply to their children at any time and anywhere.

It is based on reflexology and has been specifically designed to be an easily applied treatment for children and babies aged over one month. For thousands of years Reflexology has been recognised as a valuable and natural complementary medical treatment which requires no creams, lotions or oils and there is no need to undress the baby before treatment.

Baby Reflex has been shown to aid the wellbeing of babies; to increase the bonding between child and parent now considered as essential to early child development, and to address many other normal and worrying baby ailments and discomforts. Baby Reflex is easy and quick to learn, can aid the baby's sleep, is available for use by parents for a lifetime and can make family life during the early times after a baby's arrival less disturbed.

Working with mothers after the birth of their baby

Something I'm very passionate about and teach practitioners regularly is that when working with babies you need to treat the 'whole'. It is important to observe and listen to mum to understand the bigger picture. If mum is not well, mentally and/or physically then her baby may struggle to thrive. Baby reflexology is very much a collaboration between mum and baby, so it is vital that mum is supported, calm and present when using reflexology on her child.

Take the time to speak to mum on the phone before she attends your baby reflexology class. Ask some carefully worded, open questions, to establish how she and baby are doing. You will be able to get a sense of how mum is recovering and coping after the birth of her baby. This will allow you time to carefully plan your class to ensure that not only are her baby's needs met but you're also able to meet her needs too.

Mothers hormones have a huge impact on how they are feeling and functioning on a daily basis. We know that during pregnancy and after the birth of a baby a woman's hormones will change and fluctuate to be able to meet the needs of her baby. These changes in our hormones can, in some people, endure months after the birth of their child.

What are the signs of an hormonal imbalance and how can we support?

The main signs of an hormonal imbalance are;

- Extreme Fatigue
- Inability to lose weight
- Mood swings and anxiety
- Insomnia
- Hair loss
- Postpartum depression

When teaching practitioners I always recommend that they include a session that is purely focused on self-care for the care giver. Helping women after the birth of their baby to gain some equilibrium, and supporting them in balancing their hormones, will make a huge difference to how they are feeling, connecting and coping with the demands of being a new mum.

This can involve teaching mums some simple hand reflexology, mindfulness and breathing techniques. Taking the time in your class to demonstrate the importance of being present, working to eliminate any background noise and dedicating five minutes a day to focus solely on them and their baby.

Simple Self-Help Hand Reflexology

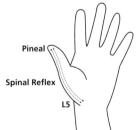

I like to incorporate breathing, visualisation and reflexology. I personally feel this brings self-care to a whole new level!

Demonstrate this technique to mum so she can pop it in her toolkit and use as and when she needs it.

Start by gently stroking down the side of the thumb, as you stroke down breathe in deeply and count in your head to three. Then stroke back up the side of the thumb, breathing out for five seconds or more. Repeat this action three times before gently placing one finger on the side of the thumb and one finger down by the heel of the hand. (spinal reflex, L5 and pineal gland).

Ask mum to hold these points, continuing to breathe steadily in and out of her nose. As she breathes, invite mum to close her eyes and begin to imagine a calm sea, as she looks out towards the ocean the warmth of the sun beams down on her face and the sea breeze gently ripples up and over her.

The visualisation can be whatever you feel is appropriate. You may want to ask beforehand if they can think of a time when they felt totally calm and relaxed. This can then be used in their visualisation if they'd prefer.

I have found the combination of reflexology (touch), breathing and visualisations incredibly powerful at eliciting a profound response with regards to calming, grounding and helping to realign the mind and body.

Breathing

How does breathing help to regulate mood and hormones?

We know that taking time to breathe slowly, helps to trigger the hypothalamus. The hypothalamus is connected to the pituitary gland which is situated in our brain. It sends out neurohormones, which inhibit stress-producing hormones and activate a relaxation response in the body. The hypothalamus is responsible for controlling and creating most of the hormones in the body and is vital for maintaining homeostasis.

Deep breathing is known to;

- Improve calmness
- Aid pain relief
- Help detoxify the body
- Boost immunity
- Increase energy
- Improve digestion

Simple breathing technique to support mums in your class or one to ones.

The breathing technique I love the most and share with my mums is square breathing. It's my favourite because we're combining touch and breath. This is great for calming an overwhelmed and flooded nervous system. Using this technique is an excellent way to start your class or one-to-one. It gives mums the time to calm and ground themselves in the present moment, which in turn will help them to focus more effectively during your class.

1. Inhale for 4 seconds
2. Hold breathe for 4 seconds
3. Exhale for 4
4. Repeat

Slowly draw a square on your hand and follow the breathing sequence.

Mindfulness

There have been many studies looking in to the effectiveness of mindfulness techniques and one recent one found that mindfulness may contribute to a mother's psychological wellbeing. **https://pubmed.ncbi.nlm.nih.gov/28173769/**

At the end of my baby reflexology classes I love to finish with a full body scan. Inviting mum and baby to snuggle up together, I start by getting mum to take in all the different noises and sounds in the room. These noises will come and go but acknowledging those sounds helps to prevent them from becoming a distraction later on in the body scan.

You can either get Mum to close her eyes or she can softly focus on her baby. Then start bringing awareness to her body and breathing.

Reflexologist script for body scan with mother:

Gently breathing in and out of the nose.

As you get comfortable start to become aware of the weight of your body relaxing in to the floor.

Get a sense of the areas which may need more of your attention. Spend a moment longer on this areas if needed.

Toes:

Send your focus down to the tips of your toes. Slowly curl up your toes, squeezing them tight and then gently release and relax, switching them off.

And breathe.

Feet:

Now moving your focus from your toes to your feet, allowing your feet to feel heavy and tired, you can feel the weight of them gently pressing in to the floor beneath you. Now switch them off.

Ankles:

Begin rotating and flexing your ankles slowly and methodically, easing out any tension or strain. Release and relax them to the floor, switching them off.

Lower legs:

Slowly move your attention to your calf muscles. Squeeze and release, letting them feel heavy and grounded, any tension gone, totally switching them off.

And breathe.

Knees:

Allow the knees to feel heavy now, imagine a warm jug of water being poured over them, helping them to relax, relieving any tension held here, before gently switching them off.

Upper legs:

Feel the muscles in the tops of your legs gently start to relax, allow the weight of them to press in to the floor and focus on switching the muscles off. Now take a deep breath in and out through your nose.

Pelvis and hips:

Sending your focus to your hips. Imagine gently rotating your hips, easing any tightness in the hip socket. Squeeze your bottom and release, letting your hips and pelvis lay heavy on the floor beneath you. Switching everything off.

Front of torso:

Start to centre your attention on your chest. Begin breathing deeply in to your torso, opening up your chest and letting the solar plexus expand outwards, creating a sense of balance and calm within your body.

Back of torso:

Imagine the back of your head and spine lengthening and stretching as you lay on the floor. Letting go of any tensions being held there.

And breathe.

Arms:

The arms can rest heavy on the floor. Imagine someone gently pressing their hands on either side of your shoulders, allow that feeling of heaviness to work its way down from your shoulders in to your biceps and forearms. Now switch them off.

Wrists and hands:

Open up your palms so they are facing towards the ceiling/sky. Gently rotate the wrists and stretch out the fingers, before allowing them to rest on the floor beneath you.

Neck:

To open up and release the neck, imagine space being created between each vertebrae, visualise this becoming wider, allowing all the tightness held here to disappear.

Head:

Imagine the head gently and fluidly pivoting on the head neck joint, allow it to become heavy and restful.

Face:

Soften the face, allowing the lips to sink down. Ease away any frowns. Relax your tongue and rest it on the base of your mouth. Create space between the eyebrows, relaxing the forehead and allowing the face to feel heavy and relaxed.

Now start to bring awareness back in to your body. Rotate your wrists and ankles. Place your arms above your head and lengthen out your legs for a full body stretch. Open your eyes and kiss your baby.

Using a range of techniques as suggested above will help to support mums and any hormonal changes they may be dealing with. This combined with teaching them baby reflexology techniques is such a powerful tool to create calm, connection, bonding and equilibrium for both mum and baby. Enjoy!

Reflexology research relevant to Baby Reflex

The three UK exploratory pilot research studies into the effects of Reflexology on child asthma, which were co-ordinated by Jenny Lee, showed some interesting results.

These three studies, set up initially to examine the effect of Reflexology on asthmatic children, took place in many centres over a wide area of the UK and Ireland and were supported and sponsored by national and medical personnel and bodies.

Oxford University; the local Watlington Hospital in Oxfordshire, an Oxfordshire Primary School, and over forty families across England, Scotland, Wales, Ireland, and the Channel Islands took part, all with The Research Ethics Committee Approval.

Every participating child was required to agree to take part in the research and the GP of each child had to agree to that patient being included.

Each family parent also had to agree to the research including their child, and a statistician was engaged to monitor and summarise the findings.

This pilot research was carried out at times specifically chosen to include the periods during which asthma is at its height, from autumn through to the winter during 1994 and 1998.

There were two very clear results from these studies.

Firstly, all the participating children receiving a Reflexology treatment, who had sleep problems or disturbed nights, experienced improvements in their sleep patterns.

In one study, which involved eight asthmatic children of varying ages, two of the youngest children, who were aged 3 and 4 years respectively, fell asleep during the 15 minutes of Reflexology treatment itself, despite that treatment being given in a hospital clinic, which is an environment more often felt by children to be far from relaxing, even hostile.

Another interesting result was that an eleven-year-old boy in one of the control groups not receiving reflexology treatment, who was himself having sleep problems at the time and before that research, particularly asked to be given reflexology as part of the follow-up at the end of the research project.

During his reflexology treatments, those professionals around, and later he himself, were all amazed that he fell asleep during his first treatment. His dislike of and inability to sleep well had clearly been overcome by his reflexology treatment.

It became clear that improved sleep, which is very beneficial and important to young children, was also of benefit to that child's parents and other family members.

Secondly was the virtually universal degree of increased bonding that took place between the child and their parents. This was recorded as taking place in most of the child groups which were having reflexology treatments in those studies.

The subsequent recognition by the medical profession of the importance of "bonding" between child and parents in early life, is now seen as an essential ingredient in early child development, and certainly adds to better relationships at home.

Some of the parents of those children taking part reported and confirmed that their children had become much nicer and better behaved to the parents themselves, after receiving regular Reflexology.

The steps that followed that research

Following on from these studies, Jenny continued her work with babies and children and began to find that parents in her working areas were very interested in learning how they might be able to give limited reflexology to their own babies and toddlers.

Those parents and mothers who used Baby Reflex techniques found that they were able to soothe and calm their babies by using the few limited baby reflexology techniques. They are easily learned.

In addition, those babies receiving such treatment from their parents usually improved their own sleeping patterns.

It had become clear to Jenny Lee that, once fully trained by a qualified baby reflexologist in certain specialised reflexology techniques, parents were soon able to safely give a reflexology treatment to their own babies with resulting benefits to the whole family.

It was after these studies that Jenny created Baby Reflex. We run courses across the UK and worldwide. For Reflexologists who are unable to attend a group course we now offer one to one online training with our Director Katie Gunn.

Jenny has since retired but her influence and the work she did to create Baby & Toddler Reflex is still the foundation of our course.

We are the original provider of Baby & Toddler Reflexology training. Our course is built upon Jenny's research findings, creating a through and comprehensive training programme for practitioners and parents alike.

If you would like to learn more about Baby & Toddler Reflex please visit our website. We provide comprehensive resources and ongoing support to all our practitioners. Information and contact details can be found on our website **www.babyreflex.co.uk**.

About Katie Gunn Bsc MAR

I'm the owner & director of Baby Reflex, I'm also a mum to three little people.

After completing my degree in Sociology, I started a career in the training and development sector. My role was to help design and deliver bespoke training packages. I was able to work with an array of different businesses and support all levels, from junior teams up to senior management. It was during this time I gained my A1 Assessing Award and later on, my Level 3 Award in Education and Training. I loved my job, but after the birth of my first child, I decided to follow a new pathway that would allow me to have more flexible working and a better work life balance.

It was whilst working full time that I decided to follow my passion for complementary therapies, and I began my training in 2007. After many years of study I gained the following qualifications:

- ITEC level 3 diploma in massage, specialising in pregnancy
- City & Guilds Sports massage diploma
- ITEC Reflexology diploma specialising in pregnancy, fertility & children and a Hypnobirthing diploma.

After training as a Baby Reflex practitioner my love and passion for supporting infants and children with reflexology was ignited.

I used all the techniques I had learnt with my own children. They responded amazingly well and loved the treatments so much, I started to realise how important these therapies are to children. I began treating lots of children locally to me and started to see positive results. With the increase in children developing mental health issues, touch is an incredibly powerful & important tool to engage and reconnect with our little ones.

I run my own clinic from my studio in Berkhamsted alongside my work for Baby Reflex. Life is busy and juggling a family of five and work commitments is often a tricky path to navigate successfully! I wouldn't change what I do for anything else in the world. Having the opportunity to combine both my love of training and reflexology has been a dream come true and I'm forever thankful.

If you have any questions please do get in touch. You can connect with me via email: **info@babyreflex.co.uk** or call me on **01442 817367**, I'm always happy to chat and offer any advice and support you may need. You can also find us on Instagram **@babyandtoddlerreflex** and Facebook **@Baby Reflex (Official)**.

Puberty –
a Child's Journey
to Sexual Maturity

by Susan Quayle of The Children's
Reflexology Programme

Puberty – a Child's Journey to Sexual Maturity
by Susan Quayle of The Children's Reflexology Programme

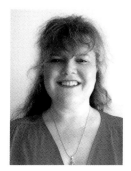

Puberty is a time of great change for children; it is the time when they start their adolescent journey into maturity and adulthood. Many changes take place throughout their body from brain development to sexual maturation and all the way through teenage angst and inbetween. It can be a time of great confusion, many, many mistakes and for some, very real trials and tribulations. In this chapter I am going to talk about puberty, what it is and how we, as reflexologists, can support not only children but also their parents and whole family unit.

Puberty is the time when children reach reproductive / sexual maturity. It is a process that can start as early as eight and continue through to age eighteen, or older. It is a time of great change and can affect every aspect of a child's life. Reflexology is a perfect tool to support your young clients during this difficult time. Little undressing is required and we can work at some distance – dealing with the feet at the far end of the body – which also allows them to completely switch off.

Many young people don't transition well into puberty for any number of reasons: low self esteem, mental health issues and depression just being a few. Reflexologists can support all teenagers with their mental health, their confusion and mindset at this difficult time by offering a clinical, nurturing attachment that has no emotional conditions placed upon them.

Just offering a space where young people can come and be themselves, without any expectation or any kind of conditions attached, will be wonderful. Having an older person that isn't a parent, and will allow them to speak openly in confidence, may offer a solid grounding foundation in their life that helps them to get through this time.

Without even using any special techniques, a general reflexology treatment is going to be very healing for them and they are going to feel so safe, enveloped in the warm embrace of a reflexology treatment room.

We have an important role that we can play in bringing these young people into adulthood whole, healthy and well, trusting in the world and their place in it. If you don't already work with this demographic, hopefully this small chapter might help you to change your mind.

Stages of puberty

Puberty has a number of stages that occur at different times, each has its own name, which occur in roughly this order.

Adrenarche

The adrenal glands begin to produce androgens which will ultimately be responsible for the production of pubic hair, oily sebaceous secretions, acne and body odour.

Gonadarche

Gonadarche can occur as early as age six but is more usual around eight or nine. The child may not be aware of any changes at this point and their body may look no different.

The body begins to produce gonadotropin releasing hormone (GnRH) from the hypothalamus deep inside the brain. GnRH is released to the pituitary gland, also located in the brain, where it stimulates the release of two more hormones: luteinising hormone (LH) and follicle stimulating hormone (FSH). LH in boys is called interstitial cell stimulating hormone (ICSH) and stimulates sperm production and secretion of testosterone from the testes.

Thelarche

Once the chemical process has begun with the release of the GnRH, everything else will follow. The first sign in girls is the development of breast buds, as the breast tissue begins to change in preparation for becoming fully functional breasts. They develop beneath the nipple area and the alveoli may start to darken too. There is an estimate of around two to four years from thelarche to the menarche, to allow for weight increase – larger girls often reach menarche earlier than those who are lighter.

Pubarche

As the androgens build, pubic hair growth will increase and hair will begin to grow under the arms too. Again it will still be a developmental process so initially thicker than before but still fairly sparse. This will increase over the coming years of puberty. Body odour, oily skin and acne will continue and a good skin cleaning routine will benefit both boys and girls.

Menarche

The menarche is a girl's first period. All girls are different and there are no absolutes in any of these phases. Girls with low body fat may feel left behind as a girl's body weight needs to be 17% fat for the menarche to occur but must be 22% for a regular menstrual cycle to be maintained.

"From the age of nine to eleven, as the body begins to make sexual changes a positive correlation was shown between a rise in leptin in the blood and BMI measurements in the child. Leptin levels continued to rise in girls but fell in boys. This resulted in girls increasing body fat in response to oestrogen and decrease in boys in response to muscle building." (Wang et al (2004))

At this point, and possibly for the next few months or years, a girl's cycle will be anovulatory, without the presence of an egg release. After the initial period she may not have another one for many months, or she may fall into a regular routine. Again there is no one-size-fits-all; we are all different.

Quick Reference Guide to Puberty Age and Observations in Girls		
Age	Stage and Phase	Observations
6+	Adrenarche	Production of androgens from the adrenal glands. These are male hormones that are present in both male and females. They drive libido, increase body hair, body odour and oily skin secretions.
8+	Gonadarche	No noticeable difference. Hypothalamus begins producing gonadotropin releasing hormone to the pituitary gland. Pituitary releases follicle stimulating hormone & luteinising hormone into blood stream.
9+	Secondary Sexual Characteristics Thelarche	Development of breast buds and the initiation of uterus growth. Some very sparse hair may start to grow around the lips of the vagina.
11+	Pubarche	Pubic hair growth increases along with underarm hair growth too.
11+	Menarche	The first period occurs. Periods may be irregular and anovulatory initially.
15+	Reproductive Maturity	Fully functional reproductive system.

Quick Reference Guide to Puberty Age and Observations in Boys

Age	Stage and Phase	Observations
8+	Adrenarche	Production of Androgens from the adrenal glands. These are male hormones that are present in both male and females. They drive libido, increase body hair, body odour and oily skin secretions.
9+	Gonadarche	No noticeable difference. Hypothalamus begins producing gonadotropin releasing hormone to the pituitary gland. Pituitary releases follicle stimulating hormone & luteinising hormone (LH) Interstitial Cell Stimulating Hormone (ICSH) in boys into blood stream.
11+	Secondary Sexual Characteristics	Testicle size increases along with the skin around them. Some very sparse hair may start to grow around the base of the penis.
13+	Pubarche	Pubic hair growth increases along with underarm hair growth. Voice breaks.
15+	Reproductive Maturity	Fully mature sexual organs

Tanner stages of growth observations

The visible stages of puberty were first observed and documented by Professor James M. Tanner, a child development expert. Today they are commonly known as sexual maturity ratings or the Tanner stages. He didn't actually put ages to the observations, simply noted the order, or stages, the developments came in and used only a series of photographs to show his observations. He observed external body developments only: breast development, pubic hair growth, penis and scrotum development.

Ages were added later for convenience.

Tanner Stage Observations in Boys		
Age	Stage and Phase	Observations
9+	1	None
11	2	Pubic hair starts to form. Testicles increase in size along with the skin around them.
13+	3	Penis gets longer. Voice starts to change. Muscles increase. May have 'wet dreams'. Growing taller.
14+	4	Genitalia continues to grow in size. Armpit hair develops. Voice deepens. Body odour and oily skin may develop.
15+	5	Genitalia has reached mature size. Hair on legs, armpits and face. Muscles are still growing. May still be growing in height.

Tanner Stage Observations in Girls		
Age	Stage and Phase	Observations
8+	1	None
9-11	2	Breast buds develop. Pubic hair starts to form.
11-12	3	Growing taller. Armpit hair forms. Oily skin & acne.
11-13	4	Breasts becoming fuller. Height growth will slow down. Pubic hair thickens.
15-18	5	Hips, thighs & buttocks fill out. Pubic hair fills out to reach inner thighs. Breasts continue to fully develop.

Reflexology to support puberty

Reflexology is a fabulous way for you to support your young clients and their parents. The general reflexology treatment that you give, along with the healing space of your treatment room and the time you are giving them, will already be of huge benefit. Never underestimate the power you give to a child when you give them the opportunity to be heard, to be encouraged to use their voice and speak their truth whilst in your room.

In the reflexology world it is well known that we are able to support clients with hormonal conditions, fertility issues, through pregnancy, right through to the menopause too. This isn't really that different except that there will need to be additional support for emotional, physical and psychological conditions that occur at this time. Going from being a child without any sexually recognisable attributes to having a body completely changed beyond all recognition, bleeding, complexion changing, hair becoming greasy, clothes not fitting, and being looked at in ways that are quite frankly embarrassing is a lot to contend with. Having a therapist that they can build a trusting relationship with, that they can confide in, who can calm them and regulate their hormones and emotions, will be a huge benefit. Having someone to talk to them about what is happening so that they are empowered will grow their confidence in their body and themselves.

Sleep may be affected at this time due to increased hormones, body changes and anxiety around all these changes taking place. Reflexology will support sleep, reduce their anxiety and help them through these challenging changes.

Always complete a full, general reflexology treatment and then add these techniques to support the endocrine and reproductive systems during this time.

These treatments, although essentially similar for boys and girls, should be given with great awareness of the intention of you, the practitioner. The work we do to support girls will be very different to that for boys, even though physically we are working the same reflexes using the same techniques and giving the same level of care. The outcomes you are looking for will be different because of the biological differences, because the emotional, physical and spiritual needs of the people that sit in front of you are very different. And this is what reflexology is about, when it comes right down to it. A set of tools that we use for everyone but is given with very personal, specific intentions for that person in front of you. This is the part that lay people don't get, they see the repetition without the beauty of the specific work involved, the years of shaping, understanding and feeling a professional reflexologist evolves as part of their mastership. The tools are the same yet they are different for every person when applied. Don't you just love our work!

Techniques

The following four techniques are the main ones I use when working with the endocrine and reproductive systems.

Balance: hold the reflex on both feet and palpate by gently pressing and releasing.

Stimulation: move your fingertips on the reflex, in a clockwise rotation with emphasis on the upward cycle of the rotation.

Sedation: move your fingertips on the reflex, in an anti-clockwise rotation with emphasis on the downward cycle of the rotation.

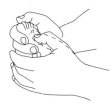

Caterpillar Walk: slide the tip of the thumb forward by extending the first joint then raise the joint to the original position by rolling the tip of the thumb in place. Repeat.

Reflexes

I know that there are many maps used within the reflexology world, these are the endocrine reflexes that I use.

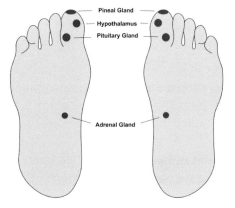

Pineal Gland
Hypothalamus
Pituitary Gland

Adrenal Gland

Endocrine Reflexes

Pineal gland: melatonin production to regulate sleep through circadian rhythms.

Hypothalamus: production of gonadotropin releasing hormone.

Pituitary gland: production of luteinising hormone & follicle stimulating hormone.

Adrenal gland: production of androgens and noradrenaline for flight, flight, freeze response.

Technique: balancing and then stimulating these reflexes will help support both boys and girls from the age of eight, or earlier. The pineal gland can help regulate sleep, which is vital to good mental health.

Reproductive reflexes

These are my reflex placements for the reproductive system.

Fallopian tubes: tubes connecting the ovaries to the uterus. They collect the released egg, which then makes its way to the uterus through these tubes. There are two, one for each ovary.

Vas deferens: ducts which connect the testes to the ejaculatory ducts for the transportation of sperm. There are two, one for each testicle.

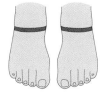

Uterus: organ for growing babies with an endometrial lining which sheds every month when there isn't a pregnancy, as part of a woman's cycle.

Prostate: gland that produces a slightly alkaline fluid that carries sperm during ejaculation.

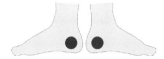

Ovaries: organs that hold eggs which develop as part of a woman's monthly cycle.

Testes: organs where sperm is produced in males.

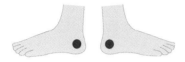

Treatments for girls

Give a general treatment followed by these:

Thelarche - 8+

Technique:
Balancing these reflexes will help support girls from the age of eight.

Endocrine balance

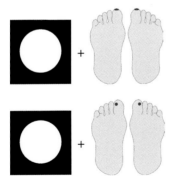

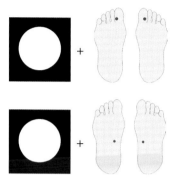

Using each thumb or a forefinger, gently palpate each pair of reflexes at a time.

Feel for changes on each side until the energy within them feels equal in both reflexes.

Reproductive balance

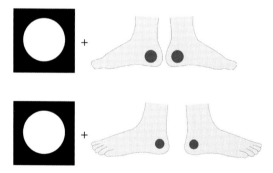

Hold each reflex to balance. Then hold the ovary & uterus reflexes of each foot to balance.

Leading up to menarche – 10+ – and after

Technique:

Balancing and then gently stimulating these reflexes will help support girls in their lead-up to the menarche from the age of ten. Good reproductive health begins with education and understanding what is happening. A girl is never too young to start taking care of her health, well-being and reproductive system.

Endocrine balance

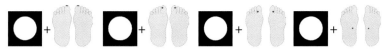

Endocrine Stimulation

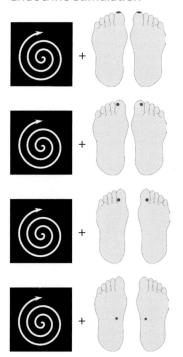

Using a thumb, or a forefinger, gently work each pair of reflexes at a time using a clockwise, circular motion. Use the palpation balancing hold to feel for changes on each side, an increase in energy is what we are looking to observe in both reflexes. Reapply stimulation until you are happy with the energy stimulation within each reflex.

Reproductive balance

Create a state of balance from which to work.

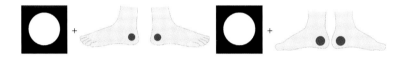

Hold each reflex to balance. Then hold the ovary & uterus reflexes of each foot to balance.

Reproductive stimulation

Stimulating the reproductive system from a state of balance allows for a more even development of the system.

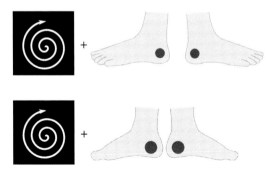

Stimulate each set of reflexes together and feel for the shift in energy. If you don't feel the energy use the palpation balancing hold to listen-feel for any changes. Reapply the stimulation technique until you are happy with the energy felt.

Fallopian tube clearing

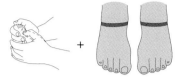

Working from above the ovary reflexes, gently caterpillar walk across the fallopian tube reflex, one at a time. Work toward the uterus reflex on the opposite ankle.

During menarche and future menstruation

Technique:

Balancing and then gently sedating these reflexes will help support girls during the menarche by promoting blood flow from the uterus.

Endocrine balance

Always create balance in the endocrine system from which to add in any extra work.

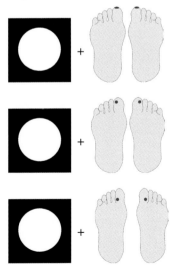

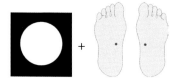

Using each thumb or a forefinger, gently palpate each pair of reflexes at a time.

Feel for changes on each side until the energy within them feels equal in both reflexes.

Reproductive balance

Create a state of balance from which to work.

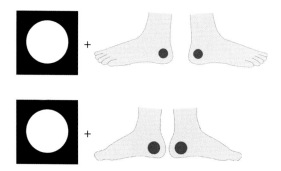

Hold each reflex to balance. Then hold the ovary & uterus reflexes of each foot to balance.

Uterus sedation

Sedating the uterus reflexes during menstruation can support blood flow from the area, helping to clear the endometrium cleanly.

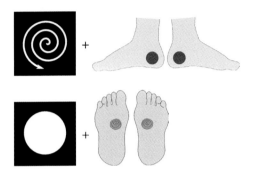

Gently sedate the uterus reflex of each foot individually. Feel for reduced puffiness in the area as you work.

Be aware that the area may be tender. If you observe signs of pain add a solar plexus hold to the treatment whilst you work the painful area and ask your client to take some deep breaths in and out.

PCOS

Polycystic Ovarian Syndrome (PCOS) is a hormonal condition that affects women. PCOS is caused by an excessive increase in the serum Anti-Mullerian Hormone (AMH) that is responsible for the development of ovarian follicles. AMH inhibits the release of Follicle Stimulating Hormone (FSH) which prevents a dominant follicle from developing and actually encourages multiple small follicles to develop instead, hence the 'string of pearls' effect on the ovary.

It has been hypothesised that high levels of AMH in utero affect the placental aromatase, which convert androgens into oestrogens in the placenta from the mother's blood and would normally prevent androgens from directing sexual development in female foetuses.

AMH levels are high when women are young and reduce with age.

Folliculogenesis

Ovarian cell development is called folliculogenesis and each egg begins as a granulosa cell. These cells take just over a year to reach full development and AMH is the hormone that facilitates this process. In women with PCOS AMH levels in these granulosa cells is seventy five times higher than in women without PCOS. So you can see why there might be a problem. AMH levels in the plasma of PCOS women can be as much as three times higher than those without it, which allows for a potential diagnosis from a blood test.

Women with PCOS have a more androgenised hormonal profile which can cause hirsutism, hair loss, weight gain and insulin resistance, skin problems such as acne as well as issues with sweat and body odour – PCOS can be a pretty hideous condition to have as a young girl about to embark on an already difficult journey. And of course it can lead to amenorrhea (no menstruation) and dysmenorrhea (painful menstruation).

Most young women who have reproductive issues are offered the contraceptive pill as a first port of call. This should be a last port of call not a first. For many women the pill adds to their problems causing migraines, acne, sickness and painful periods.

As a complementary therapist I would advocate for a longer, natural approach that works alongside the body and what is actually happening. When dealing with ovulation we need a long term plan with the view that what you start today you will be reaping in a year's time – a granulosa cell takes roughly thirteen months to become a mature egg cells are in all stages of development during folliculogenesis so things may start to improve before the year is up.

I would also ask what it is that you want to achieve. For many young women regular menstruation takes many years to reach, so this may not actually be a sensible goal to start out with. If you are suffering from the more embarrassing side effects of PCOS - excessive hair growth, weight gain, acne - and wish to try to regulate these, then creating a programme to balance the chemicals responsible for these extremes may help.

Check the diet too. The best diet for PCOS is low in carbohydrates and sugar. Eat organic meat with no added hormones or favour a vegetarian or vegan diet if you are able to. Try these ideas out and see how they work. Once out of control it is even harder for PCOS sufferers to lose weight than for others.

Treatment for control of symptoms

Teach your young clients or their daughter's to work the reproductive system themselves and to make it part of their daily self-care routine. Give a normal full treatment and then give a full hormone balance before using the sedation technique on the following reflexes:

Technique:

Endocrine balance

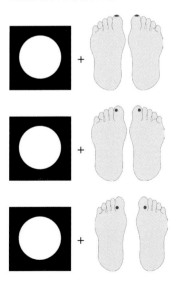

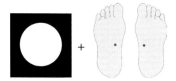

Using each thumb or a forefinger, gently palpate each pair of reflexes at a time.

Feel for changes on each side until the energy within them feels equal in both reflexes.

Reproductive balance

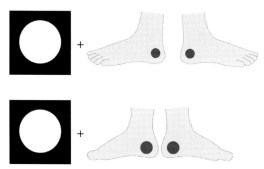

Hold each reflex to balance. Then hold the ovary & uterus reflexes of each foot to balance.

Sedating the reflexes

Pancreas

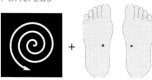

Adrenal glands

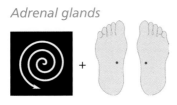

Ovaries

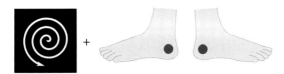

Pancreas – often an issue with PCOS especially if the client is overweight which leads to insulin resistance. If she is not overweight that's great, not all women with PCOS have all the symptoms. I would sedate it anyway though. If she is overweight, diet will be crucial to maintaining a healthy weight.

Adrenals – androgens are very active so sedation makes sense to try to control their production.

Ovaries – the AMH is active in the ovaries at a cellular level, sedation with intention is paramount, therefore I would always sedate.

Work the uterus to the normal cycle, stimulating until menstruation and then sedating to support releasing the endometrium.

Treatment for regulating the reproductive cycle

Once a young woman's cycle has reached maturity, 18 – 24 years of age, a new protocol can be used to support a regular, balanced cycle. Many women with PCOS have very long cycles, some can only bleed once a year or even longer. Reflexology can help to bring these cycles under control but it is never a quick fix.

Give full treatment followed by an endocrine balance.

Technique:

Endocrine balance

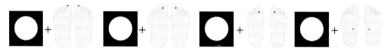

Reproductive balance

Create a state of balance from which to work.

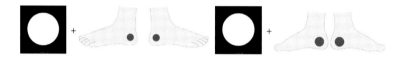

Hold each reflex to balance. Then hold the ovary & uterus reflexes of each foot to balance.

From the last day of her period begin stimulating the hormones after balancing.

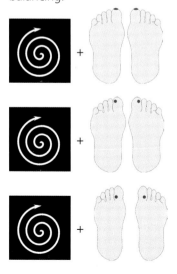

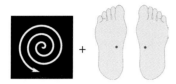

Pancreas

Apply a sedation technique to the pancreas. The pancreas can be affected by PCOS, especially if the young woman is overweight and has insulin resistance. Hyperandrogenism can cause the female body to turn energy from food into fat more readily than it would normally, creating excessive weight gain much more easily and making it much harder to reduce weight too.

Using a thumb, or a forefinger, gently work each pair of reflexes at a time using a clockwise, circular motion except the pancreas. Use the palpation balancing hold to feel for changes on each side, an increase in energy is what we are looking to observe in both reflexes. Reapply stimulation until you are happy with the energy stimulation within each reflex.

Reproductive stimulation

Continue stimulating, especially the ovaries which should be done several times a day for at least two minutes on each side, until menstruation begins.

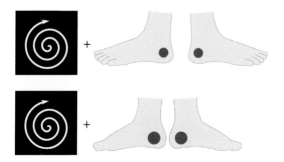

Stimulate each set of reflexes together and feel for the shift in energy. If you don't feel the energy use the palpation balancing hold to listen-feel for any changes. Reapply the stimulation technique until you are happy with the energy felt.

Fallopian Tube Clearing

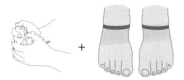

Working from above the ovary reflexes, gently caterpillar walk across the fallopian tube reflex, one at a time. Work toward the uterus reflex on the opposite ankle.

Uterus sedation during menstruation

Sedating the uterus reflexes during menstruation can support blood flow from the area, helping to clear the endometrium cleanly.

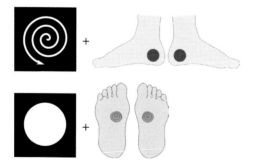

Gently sedate the uterus reflex of each foot individually. Feel for reduced puffiness in the area as you work.

Be aware that the area may be tender. If you observe signs of pain add a solar plexus hold to the treatment whilst you work the painful area and ask your client to take some deep breaths in and out.

Ovary sedation during menstruation.

Sedating the ovaries at this time may support a reduction in AMH levels prior to the release of FSH and LH. Sedating the adrenals and pancreas may help the body to balance testosterone and insulin levels.

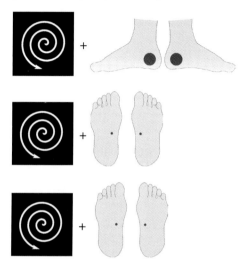

Supporting young clients with PCOS

Puberty is a very difficult time for all children but discovering that you have PCOS is going to be hard, especially if the side effects are significant. In these situations children can often go through a stage of denial, not wanting to accept big health issues when they first find out about them. Speaking to a parent can sometimes be a problem too, so having an independent, non judgemental third party can be vital, especially if they are aware of the problems being faced. Being able to share your knowledge and teach her how to help herself will empower her immediately or later when she is able to process it.

Conception

Women with PCOS are well known to have difficulties in conceiving and reflexology can really help to support them at this time, using the protocol above. However, some women may need extra help and consideration needs to be given on how PCOS is passed on through the gene pool. This information may help support your clients in relation to this.

Metformin

In research studies the drug Metformin has been shown to reduce the levels of AMH in the blood and can help to regulate the reproductive cycle. This drug is important because of its ability to reduce the AMH levels, studies have shown that she needs to take it for at least eight months leading up to conception, but as folliculogenesis is more than a year this might be preferable. Long term use requires a supplement of vitamin B12. As it is a drug given for diabetes it is actually safe to take during pregnancy. This may be a possible way to reduce the AMH levels that enter the placenta and prevent passing it on through the gene pool.

Treatments for boys

Give a general treatment followed by these:

From 8+

Technique:

Balancing these reflexes will help support boys from the age of eight.

Endocrine balance

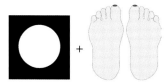

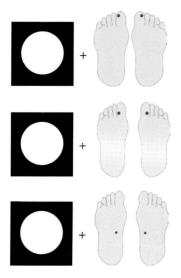

Using each thumb or a forefinger, gently palpate each pair of reflexes at a time.

Feel for changes on each side until the energy within them feels equal in both reflexes.

Reproductive balance

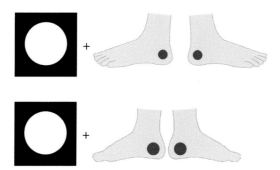

Hold each reflex to balance. Then hold the testes & prostate reflexes of each foot to balance.

11+

Technique:

Balancing and then gently stimulating these reflexes will help support boys as they start to develop secondary sexual characteristics. It will help to help them to feel safe and calm as changes begin to take place.

Endocrine balance

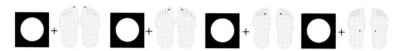

Endocrine stimulation

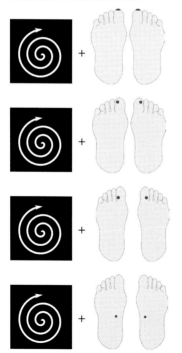

Using a thumb or a forefinger, gently work each pair of reflexes at a time using a clockwise, circular motion. Use the palpation balancing hold to feel for changes on each side, an increase in energy is what we are looking to observe in both reflexes. Reapply stimulation until you are happy with the energy stimulation within each reflex.

Reproductive balance

Create a state of balance from which to work.

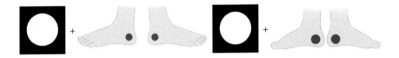

Hold each reflex to balance. Then hold the testes & prostate reflexes of each foot to balance.

Reproductive stimulation

Stimulating the reproductive system from a state of balance allows for a more balanced development of the system.

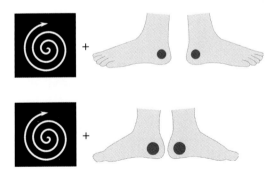

Stimulate each set of reflexes together and feel for the shift in energy. If you don't feel the energy use the palpation balancing hold to listen-feel for any changes. Reapply the stimulation technique until you are happy with the energy felt.

Vas deferens clearing

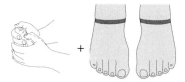

Working from above the testes reflexes, gently caterpillar walk across the vas deferens tubes reflex, one foot at a time. Work toward the prostate reflex on the opposite ankle.

Supporting parents to support their children using reflexology

In my work I am a great advocate for the empowerment of families and this is what Kids Reflex is all about: sharing this knowledge and these skills with parents to ensure that they can support their children in the safety and comfort of their own home without fear, anxiety or embarrassment. I have found that with the right approach it is possible to quickly and easily teach parents enough amazingly simple reflexology to transform their ability to help their children in trying times and daily life.

Both parents can be actively involved in a touch therapy with their children and reflexology is the most easily accessible and least embarrassing of them as only socks are taken off. It is a great time for fathers to share their own story of puberty with their sons and for mothers to do likewise with their daughters. Stories are a major part of how we learn and evolve as a species. Stories allow our children to know that they aren't the only ones going through this, everyone goes through it, even their parents, and they even turned out to be great – all children think their parents are great.

Not all girls feel a sense of pride and yearning for their menarche. For some it is a frightening time that signifies an end to their childhood, which they may not be ready to move on from. It adds to many changes that they have already noticed taking place in their body that are beyond their control and they may not like. Seeing that first bleed can be very frightening; it can be a lot of blood. It can bring huge anxiety around how they are going to deal with this every month; the mess, the smell and the discomfort are all very real and noticeable to them. Having to remember to carry sanitary products with them, having to use the toilets at school (I don't think my daughter ever used the toilet at school unless it was absolutely necessary) and just feeling like a stranger in their changing body which used to feel so familiar to them; it is a lot to take in, come to terms with and cope with.

Boys also become anxious at this time. Changes are happening for them too and there may be greater expectation on them to be manly, get involved with girls, drink or take drugs and take part in dangerous or embarrassing activities. Boys are often incredibly sensitive. I sometimes think they are actually more sensitive than girls. There is the ridiculous myth that boys have to be men and that men have to be hard, unemotional and able to take everything thrown at them. However, we know that men are, of course, only human. Boys, and men, are vulnerable to these dangerous ideologies, as indicated by the statistics for male suicide rising year upon year, and men feel they are disenfranchised within their own bodies and minds by a rule that has no truth or value to anyone.

Attachment is even more important during the teenage years than ever. As the brain begins to develop, the reward hormone dopamine requires increased stimulus to produce but the dose increases and is addictive. For this reason teenagers, and often boys in particular, begin to take greater risks than they have before. Their usual activities no longer offer a reward and they become easily bored. Their brain, still undeveloped until at least age eighteen, is unable to assess risk, yet it is rewarding them every time a risk is taken. This can get them into trouble.

If attachment is broken now, and it is natural at this age for parents to take a step back thinking their child no longer wants the same level of physical connection, it can lead to a break in attachment. Children need attachment desperately, at all ages. If they aren't getting it from their parents they will look for it somewhere else, usually amongst peers, who also have undeveloped brains, and this can lead to their inability to ever really reach maturity, as they are unable to assess risks, understand the consequences of their actions or be responsible. They are guiding each other all with, literally, half a brain. Children need to be guided in their development by adults, by parents and strong attachments are crucial in the development of all teenagers.

Due to the nature of the dopamine reward stimulus, teenagers are at the most vulnerable that they will be in their lives of addictions, suicides, accidents, pregnancies, sexually transmitted diseases and any other activity that involves dangerous risk taking, which is exacerbated by broken attachments to parents.

Having special time with mum is a healing, bonding space where children can feel held and nurtured and safe – just as they have through every other major event in their lives. There will be tears, lots of them, for any reason, and emotional explosions of anger, disappointment, fear, rage, bloody-mindedness, and just sheer stubbornness. I can tell you that the simple act of holding their solar plexus reflex in these moments will be a magical release for all the emotion that is trying to escape.

Teaching parents how to support their children using reflexology allows them to connect using the special language of love, touch and oxytocin where no words are necessary because their parent is enough, in fact their mum or dad is all they need right now. All stages of bringing up children are never really that far away from each other and this is like terrible twos on steroids (quite literally). They will always still need their mum and dad, and reflexology acts as a great leveller in the face of hormonal imbalance and emotional melt-down. It is the same story as it was when they were two; a parent grabbing their solar plexus and holding on tight until it all melts into the tears that need to flow. Then plenty of hugs, blankets, and hot chocolate while they finish the treatment. It is a special time; a rite of passage, and parents are very much needed.

This begins early; don't wait until the menarche to build this connection, parents can start today, right now. None of the reflexes here will have a negative effect when worked - it's all the body and every part of us is connected. Using reflexology will help to regulate the development of puberty over the coming years and build a trusting relationship between parents and their children, helping them to feel that they can come to their parents with any problem. This is perfect for the changing patterns that are taking place and a great way to maintain that all-important secure attachment.

You, as a therapist, can play a significant role in helping parents to support their children through this time. Yes, reflexologists are needed, but you won't be there in the middle of the night when your client's thirteen-year-old son is flipping out. Or when their daughter doesn't know what's wrong but can't be nice or happy or stop crying although she has no idea why. In these moments, reflexology is an instant game changer, it can literally dissolve these moments within seconds and re-balance a child; I have seen it done, I have done it. But that is no use to a parent without skills, without access to a reflexologist in that moment. Empowering parents with the skills required to help their family in that moment is a service you can offer them.

These are the fundamental values I offer with my Kids Reflex programme. Offering parents a small way to stay attached to their children, even as they are striving for freedom, is a great gift for the whole family.

Conclusion

Puberty is an important time in the lives of every human being. It is a time of major change and as such requires major support, from as many different places as possible. It is said it takes a village to raise a child, and puberty may well be the reason that this proverb is in existence.

We, as reflexologists, have knowledge, skills and great understanding that enables us to support this demographic in ways that parents sometimes can't. Through our kindness, the calming space of our treatment rooms, our powerful therapy and ability to give clients time and space we are able to build a strong rapport and trusted relationship that allows an individual to take the time and space needed when they are being treated by us. We can help these children through this time.

However, we have an extra service that we are able to offer to entire families. We can teach parents how they can support their children themselves and strengthen the bond between them at this difficult time.

The key to helping children through puberty is in understanding what is happening, and reflexologists can offer this knowledge to parents too. We can educate them in what to do to help their children and why. What a gift.

About Susan Quayle

Susan Quayle FFHT, ANLP

NLP Practitioner, Complementary Therapist - Specialist Maternity, Fertility Reflexologist & Children's Reflexologist.

Author of The Mouse's House & Mouse's Best Day Ever & Mouse and the Storm.

Creator of The Children's Reflexology Programme & The Children's Reflexology Programme for Additional Needs - Children's Reflexology Courses.

Empowering parents through reflexology - **www.kidsreflex.co.uk**

Award Winner in:
FHT Excellence Awards 2016 (Complementary Therapist of the Year)
Holistic Therapist Magazine Awards 2016 (Best New Business)

Federation of Holistic Therapists Accredited Course

01626 862469 - 07842 193194
www.kidsreflex.co.uk
Facebook: **www.facebook.com/pages/s/108322972519048**

Maternity Reflexology – The Basics to Treating Safely

by Association of Reflexologists,
Sally Earlam FMAR, BSc, PGCE,
(retired RGN)

Maternity Reflexology –
The Basics to Treating Safely
by Association of Reflexologists,
Sally Earlam FMAR, BSc, PGCE,
(retired RGN)

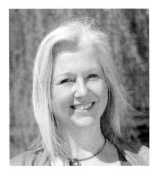

Being able to support women with reflexology throughout their pregnancy is a wonderful experience and one that we should feel honoured to be a part of. Reflexology during pregnancy aims to optimise the health of the pregnant woman and it is important that we do not treat pregnancy as an illness. Concentrate on treating any conditions that arise during pregnancy and offer support and advice accordingly. As a reflexologist we may give reflexology and general lifestyle advice, however we must not at any time give medical or obstetric guidance but rather ensure that a client with problems or concerns is in the care of the appropriate clinical practitioners.

I also believe it is important that you gain an understanding of the basic physiology of foetal development and maternal changes that happen throughout the pregnancy to enable you to talk knowledgeably to the mother. You will then be able to reassure her that what she is experiencing is normal or know when to suggest she talks to her midwife if there are concerns about her symptoms. We hope the information in this chapter will enable you to make informed decisions about working during pregnancy.

Do I need additional training to work with pregnant clients?

Most insurance companies will allow you to work 2nd and 3rd trimester, and uncomplicated pregnancies, but do check if you are unsure what your policy covers. If you wish to work with pathological pregnancies and feel you would benefit from adding to your skills and knowledge for practising safely in this area, we suggest you consider attending one of the growing number of Continuing Professional Development (CPD) workshops or courses covering pregnancy and childbirth from a suitably qualified and experienced tutor. Your course should also contain a case study element and try to find a workshop leader who will give you backup support following the course. The Association of Reflexologists (AoR) website has many AoR approved CPD courses – **www.aor.org.uk**.

Basic principles for Maternity Reflexology

As with all reflexology treatments, both the reflexologist and client must be completely happy to proceed. If there is any doubt in either's mind, then the treatment should not go ahead and be considered contraindicated. Below are some pointers though to help you make an informed choice:

- **Don't exceed your training and experience** – listen to your instinct - if you believe you shouldn't treat then don't, and seek advice.

- **Do focus on the client's health** – remember the client is not ill, they are there for relaxation and improved wellbeing. The maternity journey is one that brings not only physical challenges as the foetus grows but also times where emotional support may be required. Supporting the woman with reflexology and a listening ear can provide many benefits.

- **Know when to refer to the healthcare team** - as a reflexologist we are there in a support role and all medical care will be provided by the healthcare team. One of our main roles is to know when not to treat and when to refer our clients to their midwife, GP or consultant. If you have concerns about their health, then ask them to contact the relevant healthcare professional – they will have been given details of who to contact with concerns.

- **Do take extra care to ensure client comfort** – especially in the later stages of pregnancy, always ensure you have plenty of pillows and cushions at hand and be prepared to adapt to working in different positions and angles.

- **Don't lie your client flat in the third trimester** – this is because of the risk of supine hypotension that can occur in later pregnancy. Supine hypotension is caused if the pregnant uterus compresses the inferior vena cava when a pregnant woman is put into a reclined position, this will lead to decreased venous return.

To ensure client safety make sure that in the third trimester women are sat upright or tilted onto their left side with the pelvis tilted to 30^0 (this equates to the right hip needing to be 10-12cm higher than the left) and place cushions to keep them on their side. For those that work with Lafumas (a brand of reclining chair) this can be difficult, and you may need to think of treating the client with them sitting on a chair or sofa with their legs on a stool.

Always check that the client is comfortable and doesn't feel breathless, nauseous, sweaty or just feels panicky – in these instances sit the woman upright straight away or tilt her onto her left side to release the pressure on the vena cava.

- **Do allow extra time between ending the session and the client standing up** – feeling light-headed is fairly common throughout pregnancy even in the first trimester. High levels of progesterone relax the walls of the blood vessels, causing the vessels to dilate and blood pressure to drop. Stress, fatigue and hunger also may play a role. So always allow clients to sit for a minute or two before standing up.

- **Do research and understand your subject** – having knowledge of the pregnant state helps build your confidence and lets your clients know that they are in safe hands. If you plan to work in maternity, you could look to attend a CPD workshop/course on maternity reflexology.

- **Don't have the room too warm** – as pregnant women have a little heater inside them!

- **Do not use essential oils unless you are trained to do so** – you can use pre-blended creams and waxes but do check they are safe to use in pregnancy. Also, some pregnant women have a very sensitive sense of smell so unscented is always a good, safe bet, and turn off any oil burners or diffusers.

- **Do check if your client has had any midwife or hospital appointments and if all is progressing well**. We do not need to see their maternity notes and as reflexologists we are not able to write in the notes. Any communication with healthcare professionals should be done via the client.

Reflexology in the first trimester (0-13 weeks)

Whilst there are risks throughout pregnancy, there is a higher likelihood of miscarriage in the first 13 weeks of pregnancy. So there is statistically a greater chance that they will miscarry in the first trimester than later on in the pregnancy. This is nature's quality control in action, with the majority thought to be due to chromosonal or placental abnormalities. There is no evidence to suggest that reflexology can cause a miscarriage. Indeed, some reflexologists have seen that reflexology has been used effectively in situations where there has been a history of miscarriage, though once again, there is no research evidence to back this up, but hopefully helps to demonstrate reflexology can be a useful support in first trimester.

Some things to consider if you are planning to work in first trimester are:

■ **Check you are insured to work in first trimester** – although the AoR recommended insurance broker Alan Boswell, does cover reflexology in the first trimester, we are aware that not all insurance companies do – so do check your policy. For your reassurance, Alan Boswell have never received a claim from a pregnant client asserting that reflexology had done harm!

■ **Gain experience in treating second and third trimester maternity clients (uncomplicated pregnancies) to build your confidence**. Once you have built up your experience and knowledge of pregnancy you can start to think about treating in the first trimester.

■ **Would you worry you had done something wrong if your client had a miscarriage?** If this is the case, then do not work in first trimester yet. Once you can acknowledge that the benefit of the relaxation offered by reflexology is immensely valuable during a time when anxiety can be high, and that unfortunately some pregnancies are just not meant to be – then it is time to consider working in the early pregnancy.

■ **Would you be able to handle the communication if the women were to have a miscarriage?** If the points above have been covered then you probably would be able to deal with this situation, but it is worth thinking about.

■ **Ask clients to consent that they are happy to go ahead with treatment** - both the client and therapist need to understand and accept that there is a chance of miscarriage, especially in first trimester, and there is no evidence that reflexology causes miscarriage.

Are there any reflex points I should avoid in pregnancy?

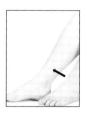

There are no actual reflex points that need to be avoided during pregnancy but there is an acupressure point called Spleen 6 (Sanyinjiao) and this should not be worked in maternity until post 37 weeks. It is found 4 fingers up from the medial maleolus (ankle bone), 4 of your client's fingers; so if your fingers are larger or smaller then it may be 3-5 of your fingers up from the malleolus on the posterior border of the medial aspect of the tibia.

It is called Spleen 6 as it is the 6th acupressure point on the spleen meridian which originates on the big toe and moves up the inside of the leg. This point, if stimulated, aims to free blood stasis from the uterus and produces a downward movement of Qi (energy), causing a contraction of the uterus and potential expulsion of the contents. You can therefore see why this point should be avoided during pregnancy.

Preparation for birth vs inducing labour

Most babies will deliver naturally by 42 weeks, but approximately 15% will need to be induced - remember though that induction is a medical procedure carried out in a hospital.

So, can we as reflexologists induce labour? Essentially no, as this is a medical procedure and what we do is much more subtle. When a client calls to ask for induction of labour, I will explain that many women find reflexology an excellent way to help the body prepare for birthing and once mum and baby are ready it can then help expediate the birth. Even encouraging relaxation at this time, when women are often worrying about the birth, can sometimes be enough for labour to start. If the body has high levels of stress hormones the body is essentially in fight or flight mode and so her body is saying – don't go into labour but run somewhere that is safe for you.

Before the induction date (usually around 42 weeks) the woman is generally offered a "membrane sweep" or "cervical sweep" which can for some women help kick start labour. Try to see the client as soon after a sweep as possible for a reflexology session as this can be quite a powerful combination!

If you have attended a maternity reflexology training course you may have learnt techniques that help prepare the body for birth or priming for birth that can be used after 37 weeks which is considered normal gestation. Whilst the premise is that reflexology will not bring on premature labour, there is no justification for using these techniques before this time. These can then help support and prepare both the body and mind for birth once the pregnancy is considered full term.

Reflexology and breech or transverse baby

Delivering a breech (or wrong lying) baby makes birthing harder and some women will be recommended to have a c-section. So, it is not a surprise that women will try almost anything to turn a baby to a cephalic position (head down).

The foetus will change position regularly during pregnancy, and this is normal. Most will settle into their final position around 34 to 36 weeks and after 37 weeks it is highly unlikely that this will change before the birth. There are many reasons why a foetus may adopt a breech presentation, and some are thought to be uterine abnormalities such as misshapen uterus or fibroids, low-lying placenta, abnormal amount of amniotic fluid or a short umbilical cord. In other words, sometimes it just is not possible, or would be dangerous for a baby to turn.

Turning a breech baby is a manual procedure known as external cephalic version, which is where an obstetrician tries to turn the baby into a head-down position by applying pressure on the abdomen. Before an ECV is attempted an ultra-sound scan is used to confirm that it would be safe for the baby to turn; the baby's heart rate is also monitored. The procedure can be very uncomfortable but around 50% of breech babies can turn.

Reflexologists should not claim to turn a breech baby as this term refers to the manual turning and it is important to differentiate this in your mind with what we do as reflexologists. There is plenty of anecdotal evidence of women whose babies have turned after reflexology and I have seen this myself. However, this is on a much more subtle level than the manual turn. The belief is that reflexology can sometimes create relaxation in the pelvic girdle and surrounding muscles and therefore creating space for the baby to turn, if it is safe for it to do so. So when you receive that call from a woman asking if reflexology can turn a breech baby my answer would reflect this last point; whilst reflexology does not actually turn the baby, sometimes by creating relaxation and space in the pelvic girdle, this will allow the baby the space to turn.

Contraindications and cautions

There are not many complete contraindications where reflexology cannot be given, however there are areas where there may be cautions. Below we have described different types of pregnancy, the medical implications and what you need to consider in terms of providing reflexology.

In all instances though, DO NOT TREAT pregnant clients

- If you feel you do not have the relevant experience, or have a any doubts
- If there are any reflexology contraindications – remember there is a higher risk of DVT in pregnancy
- If there is any vaginal bleeding – they need to seek medical help
- Sudden onset of pain - they need to seek medical help
- Severe headache, visual disturbance, indigestion like pain, very swollen feet, ankles or face or just says she feels very unwell - they need to seek medical help as these can be signs of pre-eclampsia (discussed later)
- If the woman is in hospital she will need to seek consultant agreement for her to have reflexology

Different Types of Pregnancies:

1. Uncomplicated Pregnancy

Women who are regarded as having an uncomplicated pregnancy are usually cared for by midwives either at home, in the community, at birth centres or hospital facilities.

The aim of the reflexology treatment is relaxation and to ease any symptoms or anxieties. Many women report improvements in common conditions such as constipation, heartburn, back ache, mood swings, sleep deprivation, fatigue etc. These are potential reflexology clients for all of us and the evidence is growing that having reflexology helps women through pregnancy and during the birth.

2. Uncomplicated Pregnancy plus Pre-Existing Condition

Most will have seen an obstetrician at the beginning of their pregnancy and probably will again at the end. But the rest of the care will be with the midwife in the community.

These are women who as well as being pregnant, already have a diagnosed medical condition such as diabetes, epilepsy, obesity, mental health problems (including depression and anxiety).

Medical implications – if clients have medical conditions such as epilepsy, diabetes etc. these can become more unstable for some with pregnancy.

Reflexology caution - these women can be treated by all qualified reflexologists but there needs to be some consideration of medical situations that could arise. We recommend you complete an emergency provision form which allows you to gather information as to how your client wants you to respond in the case of an emergency.

The aim of the treatment is relaxation and to ease any symptoms or anxieties.

3. Severe pre-existing condition and pregnancy

These women will have most of their care at the hospital though they may still be seen by a midwife in the community. The consultant obstetrician will be making plans for the care of the pregnancy and the birth with the parents.

Many of these women with severe disease would have been advised in the past not to get pregnant. But better health care and modern medicine have made it possible.   These are women with heart conditions, cystic fibrosis, liver and kidney disease, blood disorders such as sickle cell anaemia, uncontrolled epilepsy, hypothyroidism, severe learning difficulties and mental health problems requiring medication.

Reflexology caution - we recommend that this group of clients is treated by experienced reflexologists only who have knowledge of the condition and are able to deal with any medical emergency that could arise.

4. Pathological pregnancy, with conditions only found in pregnancy

These women will have most of their care at the hospital though they may still be seen by a midwife in the community.

The aim in maternity care is to keep women at home for as long as possible. Whilst it is fine for experienced reflexologists to treat these women if they are at home there are some considerations as there may be implications for the health of the baby and you may choose not to treat.

Pre-term labour – some of the following medical conditions do have a higher risk of pre-term labour. Whilst there is no evidence that reflexology could cause this there is evidence that high levels of stress can result in pre-term birth so our aim throughout treatments should be relaxation.

If a woman is booked in for an elective or planned caesarean section

There are many reasons why a woman may be booked to have a c-section for medical reasons when it would not be safe to have a natural birth and some conditions are discussed below.

Previously we have recommended not treating a client as her operation date approaches. This came from the reasoning that should she naturally go into early labour there may be blame placed on the reflexology. However, we do not believe that reflexology will bring on premature labour and this is a time when anxiety levels are high, and research has shown that pre-operative state anxiety may be associated with a prolonged recovery. So actually, this is a time when reducing anxiety levels could help recovery from the operation.

However, we do suggest you consider the following:

- Have you treated the woman before? – we would not recommend that you treat a new client just before her planned c-section date as you do not know how they will respond to reflexology.
- Would feel you had done something wrong if the woman were to go into labour? If the answer is yes then you should not treat.
- Consider the medical implication if the woman were to go into labour. This may include practicalities such as how far they are from the hospital that they are booked into, or if the newborn baby needs specialist care only available during normal hospital hours as compared to out of hours care.

A few common complications in pregnancy

Pre-eclampsia

Pre-eclampsia occurs in approximately 6% of pregnancies and less than 2% will be severe.

Pre-eclampsia (PE) is a disorder of pregnancy identified by the onset of high blood pressure, protein in the urine and sometimes significant swelling and this should be picked up at antenatal checks. There is no definitive known cause of pre-eclampsia, and it is thought to be related to a number of factors including abnormal formation of the placenta.

Medical implications - PE can begin after 20 weeks of pregnancy and most cases are mild and well managed. However, if it is not carefully monitored and treated it can lead to serious complications for mother and baby including seizures (eclampsia) and in some very severe cases can result in death. Whilst symptoms of PE can usually be controlled with medication the only way to cure it is to deliver the baby and this is usually around 37 to 38 weeks (induced or caesarean section), but it may have to be earlier in more severe cases.

Reflexology caution – most PE is now well managed at home with regular hospital checks. As there is potential risk to mother and baby with PE we suggest that only experienced reflexologists (who have knowledge of the medical implications, and would also be able to communicate confidently if there were medical complications with the pregnancy), treat these clients. Also encourage the client to inform her midwife that she is receiving reflexology.

The focus of the treatment is for relaxation as they are likely to be booked in to have a managed delivery. This is a time when anxiety can be high so can be a great aid to wellbeing. If the PE is severe the woman will be in hospital so she will need to seek consultant agreement for her to be able to have reflexology.

Placenta Previa (Low lying placenta) - the placenta is attached low in the uterus and may be over or close to the cervix.

Placenta Previa (PP) is usually picked up at the 20 week scan, although it may be picked up earlier as some women experience bleeding throughout their pregnancy which will prompt an earlier scan - the bleeding is caused by the position of the placenta not the caring hands of the reflexologist. However, as the uterus grows, the area where the placenta is attached often moves upwards away from the cervix and a 32 week scan will check if the placenta is still low lying.

Medical implications – if the placenta remains low at the 32 week scan, there's a higher chance that women will bleed during their pregnancy. If the bleeding is heavy it can put both the woman's and baby's health at risk. If the placenta is near or covering the cervix this can be associated with painless, bright red bleeding during the last 3 months of pregnancy, if this happens they must contact their midwife immediately. The woman will be recommended a caesarean section.

Reflexology caution – all qualified reflexologists can treat up until 32 weeks and can continue if the placenta has moved away from the cervix after this time. As there is potential risk to mother and baby if the placenta has not moved up, we suggest that only experienced reflexologists who have knowledge of the medical implications and would also be able to communicate confidently if there were medical complications with the pregnancy, should treat women with moderate to severe or grade ii to iv PP. Also encourage the client to inform her midwife that she is receiving reflexology.

N.B. If there is any bleeding this is a contraindication and they need to seek medical help.

The focus of the treatment is for relaxation as they are likely to be booked in to have a caesarean section. This is a time when anxiety can be high so can be a great aid to wellbeing. If the woman is in hospital so you will need to seek consultant agreement for her to have reflexology.

Abnormal amounts of amniotic fluid – polyhydramnios and oligohydramnios

Polyhydramnios - excessive amniotic fluid around the foetus.

Medical implications - can be linked to congenital abnormalities and risk of the cord prolapsing and becoming compressed. If it is severe this can be potentially life threatening to the baby.

Oligohydramnios – reduced amniotic fluid around the baby.

Medical implications - there is an association with both poor intrauterine growth of the baby and increased perinatal mortality, especially if this is diagnosed early in the pregnancy.

Reflexology caution – if there is mild to moderate abnormal amniotic fluid levels identified late in the pregnancy (post 37 weeks) all qualified reflexologists can treat the client. Encourage the client to inform her midwife that she is receiving reflexology.

If this is diagnosed in second trimester the risks of foetal mortality are high and the client should only have reflexology from experienced reflexologists who would be able to cope and support the woman if she were to lose her baby. If it is severe the client may be in hospital and should only be treated with consultant approval.

The focus of the treatment is relaxation and to ease any symptoms or anxieties, although there is anecdotal evidence that amniotic fluid has improved with reflexology, but there is no research evidence to back this.

Obstetric cholestasis or intrahepatic cholestasis

Obstetric cholestasis (OC) affects 1 in 140 women and is a disorder that affects the liver during pregnancy. This causes a build-up of bile with the main symptom being itching of the skin, especially palms of the hands and soles of the feet, with no skin rash. In rare cases a woman may develop jaundice. The cause of obstetric cholestasis is not yet understood, but it is thought that hormones, genetic and environmental factors may be involved and this will disappear after the birth.

Medical implications – the effects of OC on the baby are still not clear but there appears to be an increased chance of a premature birth (1 in 10 women with OC will have their baby before 37 weeks although this does include women who have their labour induced). There was also a small research study many years ago which suggested there was a higher risk of stillbirth. However, recent research has shown that the rate of stillbirth with women with OC is now the same as the normal population (this may be because of improved antenatal care).

Reflexology caution – most women with OC will be at home having regular antenatal checks, potentially daily. They are likely to be booked for a caesarean after 37 weeks, with 10% needing preterm delivery. We suggest that only experienced reflexologists who have knowledge of the medical implications, and would also be able to communicate confidently if there were medical complications with the pregnancy, treat these clients. The focus should be on relaxation which in turn can bring about improved blood flow. If the woman has jaundice, remember there is already a build-up of toxins in the body so work gently to not overload the body. Also encourage the client to inform her midwife that she is receiving reflexology.

History of premature birth.

Babies are usually born between the 37th and 42nd week of pregnancy. Those born before 37 weeks are regarded as premature. The reasons as to why some babies come very early remains a mystery. However, they are aware that for some, it can be to do with infection as early administration of antibiotics in these circumstances appears to help the baby's survival.

If a woman has had a previous premature birth she is more likely to have one again with subsequent pregnancies.

Medical implications – premature babies, especially those born very early, often have medical problems including: low body temperature due to a lack of stored body fat, laboured breathing or respiratory distress and a lack of reflexes for sucking and swallowing, leading to feeding difficulties. Premature babies will be taken to special care. If a woman has had a previous premature birth she will be carefully monitored and likely to have antibiotics during the pregnancy.

Reflexology caution – if a client has had a previous premature birth, then only experienced reflexologists who understand that this client is more likely to have a premature birth in this pregnancy due to her medical history and are able to communicate confidently with women that there is no evidence that reflexology causes premature labour but has benefits with relaxation and symptom control, should treat these clients. Also encourage the client to inform her midwife that she is receiving reflexology if the client is in hospital and she should only be treated with consultant approval.

Supporting the maternity journey

We trust that this information will prove useful for you in supporting and treating pregnant clients. This is only a guide so don't lose sight of your intuition. It is better to be cautious when treating pregnant women and don't feel afraid to say that you are unsure and/or to seek advice.

Enjoy your treatments of pregnant women. It is a very special time and is a great journey to be able to be with them through all the ups and downs, and then hopefully to be able to share their joy at the end when you finally see mother and baby together.

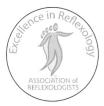

At the Association of Reflexologists we pride ourselves in providing information and support for our members. You can find out how to become a member of our reflexology community by visiting our website **www.aor.org.uk**

Chinese Medicine and Pregnancy Reflexology

by Heidi Armstrong

Chinese Medicine and Pregnancy Reflexology
by Heidi Armstrong

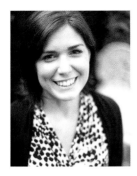

The modality of Reflexology works really with the theory base of Traditional Chinese medicine (TCM). It links energy or Chi which governs the day to day energy and health of a person, and the Essence or Jing which governs growth cycles from puberty, reproduction to menopause and can give us a unique perspective to support our clients.

The Chi and Jing help regulate the mental, physical, emotional and developmental aspects of the organ systems of the body, which are beautifully represented on the organ map of feet. This gives us a perfect system to be working Chinese medicine through reflexology.

Essence (or Jing)

It is the substance that underlies all organic life and is the source of organic change. It is thought of as fluid-like, is supportive and nutritive and is the basis for reproduction and development. It has two sources – prenatal (derived from parents' energy at the time of conception) and postnatal (mainly derived from food).

It is stored in the kidneys and the extraordinary vessels. We can think of Jing as our constitutional energy, our DNA, our reproductive hormones. It is said to flow in 7 year cycles in women and 8 year cycles in men. In a simple way through supporting the kidneys, CNS and endocrine systems in Reflexology we support the clients' Jing and all stages of growth and development.

Chi

Chi (Ki or Qi) is life's animating force. It is the creative or formative principle. It is invisible and is understood in terms of the effect that it produces. There are several forms of Chi in humans - original Chi is derived from the essence, transmitted by parents at the time of conception, has a fixed amount and can be preserved but not replenished. The Chi we produce ourselves is derived from Air Chi (is derived from the breath) and Food Chi (is derived from the food that we eat.)

Eastern perspective on pregnancy

Even though within original texts of Chinese medicine, information on pregnancy and gestation is often not clear or consistent. It was clear however, that the Chinese considered pregnancy to be an important time in a woman's life, as there are big changes in her energy, and this is felt to offer the possibility of positive change.

A woman's health can be strengthened through pregnancy. Of course, it could be a drain on the mother's energy, this is more likely to be the scenario if the mother was in poor health at the time of conception or is under stress and overworked during pregnancy.

Pregnancy is defined as 10 lunar months. It is seen as being predominantly a time of Yin energy therefore energetically, women do tend to want to move inside themselves and focus on their growing baby.

Pregnancy as a state of Yin/Water

At conception, Yang is the sperm, which provides the spark of energy to begin the process of transforming the Yin egg into the embryo. Pregnancy is about the development of a material being and takes place in the watery environment of the womb –Yin energy in relation to conception and birth. The cessation of menstruation means that more Blood energy is available, mirroring what we know physiologically about the maternal increase in blood volume. Blood energy and body fluids are part of Yin fluids. Following the movement of the five elements, water is considered the state from which we come. The baby is nourished, especially in the first trimester by the mother's essence – which is stored in her kidneys.

For all these reasons, pregnancy is considered to be a Yin state.

Yang aspects of pregnancy

Yin cannot exist without Yang. The absence of periods leads to an accumulation of fire heat in the body and heat needs to be supplied to the foetus. This is how the Chinese viewed the rise in core body temperature in pregnancy.

During pregnancy there are more of all energies, Yang included.

If there is insufficient Yin, this can exasperate excess Yang energy, which tends to rise. Excess Yang rising is the basis of the energetics behind migraine and even pre-eclampsia. So, overall supporting of the mother's energy and the balance of rest and movement are important.

Mother and child interactions: foetal education

The foetus is seen as fully formed by the end of the 3rd month and the concept of "foetal" education (Tai Kyo) is very important from this point onwards. Foetal education is where they saw the development of the foetus being on all levels emotionally, spiritually and psychically. It is said that ideally the mother should be surrounded by positive, calm energy, eat good foods, have a balanced emotional and physical lifestyle to support the baby's whole development.

We see how this has become backed up in western science with the growing knowledge and understanding of the effect of maternal stress or poor nutrition on the environment in the womb and how this can affect the baby throughout the rest of its life.

Dominant meridian for each month of the ten lunar months of pregnancy

As Chinese medical theory has developed each developmental stage for mother and baby, conditions and pathologies in pregnancy have been related to different organs/meridians and elemental theories. As these each go into great detail, I have chosen to expand on one that can help us support the harmony throughout the pregnancy.

Over the centuries a theory has developed, which refers to patterns of dominant organ/meridian energy in the mother, which nourishes the baby during the different months. These dominant meridians do not necessarily directly correspond to the 5-element theory of each trimester.

It has been said that some schools used to say that the dominant meridian for the mother in the month should not be worked. This is not considered relevant advice today but seen as important to support the mother's energy focus during the different months, as if these do not support the foetus properly, they could cause developmental issues in the corresponding organs in the baby.

Working with these ideas can help us to support the harmony and natural flow of the pregnancy.

First month – Liver - represents the beginnings of creation. Blood gathers in the Uterus. The liver stores the blood and is responsible for the smooth flow of blood. It is suggested that the mother rest in order to support the blood gathering in the uterus. Our focus is to work gently with lots of linking and holds to support the settling of the energy. This is also why we avoid using the acupressure point liver 3 (during the whole of the 1st trimester) as it promotes too much movement of blood.

Second month – Gall Bladder (GB) – this represents the movement of blood as it continues to gather in the Uterus. We continue to support this focus as in first trimester. This can also relate to the release of relaxin as the GB relates to joints, so even though there are not many postural changes, there may start to be more joint instability even in the first trimester.

Third month – Pericardium Heart protector – completes the action of enriching the blood with the Spirit. It is at this point the foetus is considered to exist. We can support the heart connection with the baby here by linking the heart and the uterus reflexes, using holding or linking techniques to support the heart and emotional connection with the baby, and encouraging the mother to use visualisations to connect to the baby.

Fourth month – Triple Heater – this continues the process of Blood moving through the body and the continued development of blood and blood vessels in the baby. It is also about the movement of water, fluids and moving Ki through the body.

Working lymph reflexes and peripheral circulation will support this process for mother and baby.

Fifth month – Spleen/ pancreas – the mother's blood nourishes the growing baby as it lays down more fat. Encouraging the Mother to ensure she has good nutrition and supporting the mother's spleen and pancreas reflexes.

Sixth month - Stomach – continues the giving of nourishment to baby. However, it is considered important in this month that the mother does not eat too much food. This is often the month that the mother may begin to experience heartburn and does need to start to eat smaller amounts of food, maybe at more times through the day. We can focus on the movement down through the digestive system to ground the stomach energy.

Seventh month – Lung energy develops. We often see mothers getting more breathless at this stage as this energy is drawn on more. Supporting the mother's breathing patterns and releasing the diaphragm is very helpful here.

Eighth month - Large intestine is paired with Lungs. Breathing of the mother is considered especially important during these last months. The large intestine is processing meconium and ready to be able to let go of waste after birth.

Ninth month - Kidney- preparing the baby for the completion of the ancestral plan. Supporting the kidney energy is vital here. Linking of pituitary and adrenals is great for this.

Tenth month – Bladder – the Yang aspect of water, preparing for birth. We can support the spinal reflex (this has links to bladder meridian) and work it towards the sacrum as the Yang energy needs to build here to be able to go into labour.

By working with the mother's organ system during her pregnancy, we are supporting two people to grow to their full potential. It is a very important time to work and is seen to support the constitution of the baby for the rest of its life.

Heidi Armstrong ARM FSS runs Complementary Therapy College and teaches "pregnancy linked to Chinese medicine" to reflexology, massage and shiatsu practitioners.

Her website is **https://www.complementarytherapycollege.com**

My Approach to Fertility Reflexology, with Naturopathic Support

by Dorothy Kelly

My Approach to Fertility Reflexology, with Naturopathic Support
by Dorothy Kelly

BSc (hons) Cert Nat DiEAT DPCM MAR

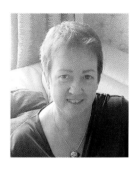

The naturopathic approach to health concentrates on whole patient wellness, while emphasizing prevention and the process of self-healing through the use of natural therapies, such as:

- Nutrition
- Herbal Medicine
- Acupuncture
- Homeopathy
- Hydrotherapy
- Physical Manipulations
- Colonic Irrigation
- Iridology
- Fasting
- Bach Flower Remedies
- Reiki
- Emmett Technique
- EFT
- Exercise

We, as therapists, are trying to bring back balance to the fertility client, through working on reflexes such as endocrines or reproductive reflexes, by trying to regulate the cycle or supporting those clients with PCOS or endometriosis, with unexplained fertility problems, blocked fallopian tubes, and for those using donor eggs or sperm for example.

Couples on this journey will come from different walks of life, be they heterosexual or homosexual partnerships, health aware or unaware, who are seeking support and guidance. It is up to us as therapists to provide our experience and support, using the tools we are qualified to use. Within this article I will discuss some of the approaches I use or signpost to clients. I have a network of therapists I engage with, including homeopaths, herbalists, nutritionists, Emmett Technique Practitioner or other fertility reflexologists if distance of travel is problematic. I think it is important for all therapists to build a network of therapists with other modalities who can work together to support each other when necessary.

There are many female pathologies which may affect fertility, such as:
- Anovulation (failure to ovulate)
- Amenorrhea (absent periods)
- Oligomenorrhea (scant periods)
- Menorrhagia (excessive bleeding)
- Fibroids (benign tumours of the myometrium)
- Pelvic inflammatory disease (PID)
- STIs, salpingitis, ovarian cysts
- PCOS
- Endometriosis, hormonal imbalances causing low progesterone or luteal phase defect
- Oestrogen imbalances
- Abdominal surgery causing adhesions

Some of the male pathologies which can affect male fertility are:
- Infections of the epididymis and testis
- Orchitis
- Hydrocele
- Prostate infections
- Impotence

- Erectile dysfunction
- Poor, no or low sperm count
- Motility or morphology of sperm

Fertility can be affected if there are problems with delivering the sperm from the testes. Problems anywhere along the tract from the testicles, including the epididymis, vas deferens, and prostate, can affect fertility.

Retrograde ejaculation — when the ejaculate goes in the wrong direction — can decrease fertility, though not necessarily sperm count (there are new innovative ways to combat this failure, such as Surgical Sperm Retrieval using Micro-Tese in the testes for retrieving sperm, or from the epididymis using either PESA or MESA). This includes immotile sperm that are alive and healthy – Kartagener's Syndrome – these sperm can be removed and injected into eggs in order to fertilise them.

Use of medication such as Tamsulosin can cause no ejaculate to be produced.

Sexually transmitted diseases can affect the fertility of the male or female and there is a growing number of chlamydia sexually transmitted infections (STIs) recorded throughout the UK, among other STIs. Generally this STI doesn't cause any symptoms, but if left untreated, the infection can spread to other parts of the body and lead to long-term health problems, such as pelvic inflammatory disease (PID) in females, epididymo-orchitis (inflammation of the testicles) and infertility. It is passed on through unprotected sex (sex without a condom). However, this STI can be treated using antibiotics.

This is why I complete a detailed consultation, to ensure that I have the full facts about the couple, including their sexual health and if needed, I can refer them to other therapists, or for further investigations. There will be discussion of some of these conditions throughout. Some will require surgical intervention but the foundation, from a naturopathic perspective, is to use an eclectic approach to meet these challenges and guide clients back to vibrant health.

The joy of bringing new life into a family, whether conceived naturally or through donor, be it egg or sperm, is an uncertain journey over variable terrain. From the client, as the one who chooses to nurture this embryo through the various stages of development, to the baby who is the most precious and yearned for child, it is a magical experience to be a part of.

The key to creating the optimum child starts way before conception

Preparation and planning for pregnancy should begin at least 3–4 months prior to trying to conceive. Any egg that your client's body releases at ovulation has been maturing in the background for around 120 days, while sperm cells need about 72 days (two and a half months) to be created, mature, and get ejaculated. It often takes that long to also see improvements in the count and the couple will want the health of both egg and sperm to be top notch. This is the typical amount of time for egg and sperm maturation.

The optimization of both parents' health will improve chances of healthy egg and sperm development, which often increases the odds of healthy conception and a successful pregnancy. I tell my clients that this approach typically takes a minimum of three to four months and offer guidance towards this in my booklet, which I give to each client at the initial consultation. (Email me at: **dorothykelly59@ gmail.com** I'm happy to send you a digital copy of my booklet upon payment of £8 fee via PayPal or BACS.) Each client/couple are told at the outset that this journey is not a quick fix, that they have their role to play and that it will take as long as it takes, or it will continue until they make the decision to bring it to a conclusion, in conjunction with myself. I recommend initially that we work together for 12 weeks and review results at this point. Other tools which I may include in the treatment process are meridians, chakras, naturopathy, womb massage, and reflexology, whilst other modalities such as herbs, homeopathy Emmett and Bowen Techniques and acupuncture can also be introduced.

If clients have already had their hormone profiles completed along with progesterone blood tests, I am keen to read the results. The hormone profile, when performed within the NHS, consists of LH, FSH, Prolactin and Oestradiol. Progesterone must be requested separately since it is not generally performed as part of the profile, as it is an expensive test. Private laboratories may also include thyroid function test and/ or thyroid antibodies. However, the antibodies will not be performed by the NHS unless the GP has a clinical reason to do so, as it is another expensive test. The use of a recent test results for both the male and female, can be used for comparison as a before and after outcome. Showing, via test results, where improvements have been made after changes have been implemented by the clients, develops a much more evidence-based form of practice, which can be demonstrated as clear medical outcomes. Causal factors for fertility represent approximately 30% female, 30% male and 30% joint conditions.

The male partner should have a semen analysis (SA) performed. Those SA's performed in the local hospital laboratory, particularly in Northern Ireland, will contain the basic information required of such a test:

- Volume
- Motility
- Morphology
- Concentration
- Total sperm

Those clients who attend our locally established private SA testing Laboratory (Examen), established by Prof Sheena Lewis, (previously known as 'Sperm Comet') will provide a much more informative report. 'Examen' specialises in measuring sperm DNA fragmentation (known as sperm DNA damage) to help predict the likelihood of conception, miscarriage and the success of fertility treatment. 80% of the UK's leading fertility clinics use 'Examen' but the NHS in Northern Ireland does not!   It is forgotten that there could be a hormonal problem or a chromosomal defect to male fertility such as low testosterone levels, FSH levels or a chromosome abnormality such as Klinefelter syndrome. This syndrome is a sex chromosome disorder in boys and men that results from the presence of an extra X chromosome in cells. This condition may not become apparent until the couple are trying for a baby, as this results in sterility of the male partner. The use of a sperm donor or ICSI may be offered as an option to the couple.

Testosterone is necessary to keep the male reproductive system working properly. Maintaining normal concentrations of testosterone promotes spermatogenesis. The hypothalamus and the pituitary gland in the brain integrate external and internal signals to control testosterone synthesis and secretion and are, therefore, areas to assess when performing reflexology.

Preparation

Preparation and planning involve numerous aspects of the individual/ couple. From a naturopathic approach, gut health is the most important aspect. Good gut health supports the assimilation of nutrition to feed the body through organic fresh foods, beneficial fresh water, supplementation and probiotics such as kefir or kombucha, which in turn build and support the immune system and encourage the growth of good gut bacteria. A strong population of a wide range of strains of probiotics also helps to clean the bowel and strengthens the enteric brain. There will be beneficial knock-on effects for the whole body.

Proper detoxification accompanied by balanced hormones and gentle exercise such as walking in nature, yoga or pilates, or quietening the mind with meditation all help.

Detoxification

Another aspect of health and hormonal balance comes down to the status of the liver. The liver detoxifies many substances such as caffeine, alcohol, drugs, pesticides, other environmental toxins, food additives, preservatives and toxins produced from bowel bacteria. To support and boost your liver function it is beneficial to undertake a liver detox every 6 months preferably, or at least once yearly. It will give your liver a rest and can be done for anything between 8, 10 days or over a longer period of 30 days if you wish a more gentle process. Regardless of the length of the process, there are guidelines of what foods and fluids can be consumed and the foods or beverages which must be avoided, to ensure an effective detoxification of the systems. Detoxification can be performed using specific herbs or homeopathic kits. It is especially useful for those clients who have recently had a treatment cycle of IVF or ICSI for example, by helping the liver break down the build-up of hormones and remove the metabolites of the chemicals consumed.

 Another avenue worth considering is the status of the colon. We in the west, unfortunately have tendency to develop 'dirty colons' over time. This is largely due to our diet and low water intake. A dirty colon will lead to autotoxication, as years of impacted faecal and mucoid material take up permanent residence on the colon wall. We absorb a great deal of water through the colon, so if we are absorbing it through putrefying material, it does not do our system much good. To go the extra mile in preparedness of the body, a bowel cleanse is seriously worth considering. It involves a detox and a herbal preparation to be taken over 10 days and it will strip off all the impacted mucoid material and all the bad bacteria which has taken up residence along the whole digestive tract.

Of course, you will need to take probiotics for a protracted period after the cleanse, before the bad bacteria get a foothold in the new clean environment. Kefir and/or kombucha are probably the best ways of getting a really broad spectrum of species into your gut. To avoid a future build up, you should remove/reduce mucoid forming foods from the diet. These include white flour products, dairy products, red meat, eggs and any foods which irritate your bowel. The bowel cleanse kit can be obtained from **www.blueherbs.co.uk**.

Lifestyle and diet

Dietary habits need to be examined thoroughly for both parties:

- What is their intake of fast foods and processed foods?
- Do they regularly make meals from scratch with wholesome and fresh vegetables?
- Do they know the benefits of organic food and are they prepared to engage with it to optimise their treatment outcome?
- Do they drink enough plain water & herbal teas?
- Are they aware of their alcohol & coffee intake & the effects of overindulgence on the likelihood of treatment success?

There must be an examination of their lifestyles:

- Sedentary or active
- Are they under- or overweight
- What are their stress levels like? Are they related to occupation or otherwise? Can they be addressed?

All areas which impact your client(s) functioning optimally within the four Naturopathic Tenets of Physical, Mental, Emotional & Spiritual.

Ideally clients should make their food from scratch using wholesome, organic fresh vegetables and drinking non-carbonated, good quality water. Salad vegetables (alfalfa is a good source of minerals and chlorophyll), berries, seeds and nuts are good for maintaining blood sugar and hormonal balance, alongside hearty and wholesome soups, and vegetable curries/stews for those whose first love isn't vegetables as they can be easily disguised.

Some things to avoid and some things to embrace

Garden peas should be avoided for those on their fertility journey, as they contain **m-xylohydroquinone** which acts as a natural contraceptive. For those men who consume these, it has been shown to reduce sperm counts by 50%. This research is not recent but I think it's worth acknowledging it, so much so that peas can be removed from the diet without causing too much heartache and why not, if your client is trying so hard to achieve this longed for baby.

Soybeans – they disrupt your ability to get pregnant. It has to do with their high content phytoestrogens; the egg production and ovulation is affected by excess intake of oestrogen which leads to a hormone imbalance.

Phytoestrogens – this is a topic I like to discuss with the client. **Phytoestrogens** have been shown to have both **oestrogenic** and **anti-oestrogenic** effects and are found in plant-based foods. This means that, while some **phytoestrogens** have **oestrogen**-like effects and **increase oestrogen** levels in the body, others block its effects and decrease **oestrogen** levels. A quick google search will reveal a comprehensive list of vegetables having both effects.

Generally, the benefits of including these phytoestrogen-rich foods in your diet outweigh any potential health risks. Favourable foods are: garlic, flax seeds, sesame seeds, dried fruits (sulphur free) cruciferous vegetables etc.

My main concern is to do with the artificial phytoestrogens: **Xenoestrogens** that the client is exposed to, such as those found in:

■ Water (tap water, bottled and bathing) – raise the question of the quality of tap water, or ask clients to think about the length of time a bottle of water has been on its journey to reach the shop shelf? How long has it been sitting in a warehouse, or has it been exposed to direct sunlight during this time? How fresh is it in reality?

- Pesticides, herbicides and insecticides - preservatives found in foods, including glyphosate as found in conventional food, and even tampons. It is good to wash all foods before we use them, using either apple cider vinegar or effervescent vitamin C tablets. It is best to use organic, which will be free of these contaminants. There is a strong argument for the case that most vegetables are impossible to be completely free from pesticides.

- Cleaning products - (home and industrial) contain many toxic substances. It is worth sourcing products free of these substances.

- Personal products – many deodourants contain a combination of perspiration/deodorant chemicals which have been found to have a link to fertility and cancers. Chemicals are parabens, triclosan, phthalates, propylene glycol and aluminium. Always ensure it is a deodorant used rather than anti-perspirant which is absorbed by the body via your armpit and may also block the pores, preventing your skin from eliminating properly, locally resulting in toxins. Consider a more natural and/or organic product. Forms of Soap can also be a contentious item. Better to seek out vegan forms, free of palm oil and made using a cold press process. Conventional tampons and sanitary towels are bleached with whitening agents containing dioxins, dyes, perfumes, pesticides which play havoc with the body's natural secretions and flora. Say 'no' to douches and feminine wipes which again destroy the body's natural barriers and flora. I suggest to clients to take a probiotic to encourage vaginal health – the good bacteria which is needed continually to provide balance and a healthy environment. A properly balanced environment in the vagina ensures that it cleans itself naturally.

- Plastics (food, beverages, storage containers, non-food packaging and industrial plastics) - many leach chemicals into the packaged food which are then consumed.

- Canned foods - I'm keen to discover what kind of non-food packaging that clients use and the wrappers they use for storing food in the home. I try to encourage the removal of cling film, Styrofoam used as food trays, aluminium foil for wrapping food and Teflon coated cooking utensils, as all of these can be harbours of xenoestrogens. Once you get these artificial hormone disruptors into the body, they can be difficult to remove and cause hormonal imbalances in both the male and female. Once clients become aware of such information, they can start to clean up their diet and dispose of chemically loaded house cleaning products, to support their cleaner lifestyle. If a client is concerned about mineral overload, they can obtain a mineral hair analysis which can show if there is heavy metal poisoning. If results show there is an overload, clients are offered detoxification instructions or they can use supplementations such as Chorella or Spirulina, following a strict dose regimen with added liver support.

- Medication and drugs that can affect fertility - recreational drugs (marijuana and cocaine) lower sperm counts. Cimetide (Tagamet), ranitidine (zantac) stomach preparations can lower sperm counts or produce impotence. Blood pressure medication can play havoc with erections too. Tamsulosin and Finasteride will prevent ejaculation in most men.

MEDICAL CONDITIONS affecting fertility can include: diabetes, lupus, cancer, coeliac disease.

Supplementation

The use of supplementation is another important aspect of preparing for conception.

ASTAXANTHIN – a carotenoid found naturally in algae consumed by marine life like shrimp, lobster and salmon, works by improving blood flow. For men, it can improve sperm count and motility. In women, it's been considered for its properties as a protective antioxidant, that can keep healthy eggs from being damaged before they are fertilised and implanted.

FOLIC ACID – this should be started 3 months before conception, to help levels build up in the tissues. Folic acid is important in the early weeks of a developing baby, which is why it is taken during pregnancy, but it can also help improve egg quality before conception. The best form to obtain for optimal absorption is **5-MTHF** - it is the natural form of folate B9. It is the bioavailable form of folate and is the only type able to cross the blood-brain barrier. It is found in food such as leafy green vegetables. It is already active and ready for the body to use. The company **BioCare** is a good source of these supplements **www.biocare.co.uk**.

HEALTHY FATS - a high intake of polyunsaturated fats has been shown to improve pregnancy rates. Try to increase intake of avocados, nuts, seeds, fish and olive oil. Some women also take a fish oil supplement - one type of fat called DHA is thought to help support brain development when a child is in utero. The best form is cold pressed oil, rather than an oil from the liver of the fish, as the liver is likely to contain toxins.

IODINE – deficiencies in this can cause an array of conditions, some being those to do with female fertility and thyroid disorders. Iodine needs its cofactor selenium to work effectively in the body. Selenium will protect cells against free radical damage and helps protect the thyroid against excess iodine exposure but should be monitored by a qualified practitioner.

L-CARNITINE – an amino acid produced by liver and kidneys. When low, it has been linked to infertility in men. As a supplement it has been considered to address age-related fertility in females and should be used alongside CoEnzyme Q10.

PRENATAL NUTRIENTS - any standard prenatal should contain a mix of B12, iron, zinc, selenium and vitamins A, C and E. Studies show better egg health and pregnancy outcomes when clients take a full prenatal, instead of just folic acid. There are specific brands that I suggest to clients. I do not recommend 'Pregnacare' as it is synthetic. The product I do recommend is 'Fertility Plus for Women' or Proxceed which is also available for male and female clients and can be purchased on Amazon.

VITAMIN D - many women are deficient in vitamin D, and studies suggest that adequate levels support better quality embryos and increase chances of a healthy pregnancy. It can be useful to get levels tested to see how much the client should be taking but generally, GPs don't encourage this unless you have significant symptoms of deficiency, as the test to the NHS is expensive and the laboratories only perform this when they have large batches of requests. If this is something the client is keen to have performed, there are private Laboratories who will perform this test, such as **York Test - www.yorktest.com** who will provide a 19 marker test, which includes vitamin D among other levels. This requires a pinprick blood test which the client then returns for processing. Results are returned to the client with a clear and easy to understand explanation.

Supplementation when preparing for pregnancy is important, but nutritional choices should not be forgotten either. Brand choice is equally important as cheaper products may not necessarily provide the optimum daily dose. The cheaper brand may consist of synthetic nutrients rather than natural nutrients. The body will then metabolise and absorb less of the daily dose than if a more expensive natural brand is purchased. Coupled with this is the need for a diet diverse in fruits and vegetables, balanced with whole grains and healthy proteins to help support blood sugar levels, combined with a healthy lifestyle, to make the best egg and sperm possible for the couple. Every client receives a list of foods and their nutritional value from me, to help them with their healthy choices when making meals.

Consultation form

There are many areas within the consultation form where I require greater detail, and I will comment on these as we go through this discussion.

Dorothy Kelly, Fertility Reflexology ©
Fertility Consultation Form

Name:	DOB:
Address:	GP:
Tel:	Email:
Occupation:	Stress Levels (score 1 -10, 1 good,10 bad) Score:
Your weight:	Age of menstrual onset:
Do you smoke:	Regular: Not regular
Units of alcohol weekly:	Cycle frequency: / days
	Aware of ovulation: Pain:
Consistency of bleed: Spotting: Beginning ☐ Mid cycle ☐ Length of period: No: days: _____	Colour of bleed: Bright red ☐ Brown ☐ Dark red ☐ Clots ☐ Intermenstrual bleeding ☐ Excessive bleeding ≥ 1 pad/tampon per hour ☐
Smear history: Up to date: Yes/No Normal: Yes/No Abnormal: Yes/No	Referred for Colposcopy: Yes/No If Yes, result CIN 1 ☐ CIN 2 ☐ CIN 3 ☐ Any further follow-up required: Yes / No
Painful periods or crampy? Yes / No	Painful Ovulation? Yes / No
PCOS ☐ Endometriosis ☐	Fibroids ☐ Cysts ☐
Low backache ☐ Other backache:	Frequent urination ☐ Frequent UTIs ☐ Thrush ☐
Cervical Mucus: Yes / No	Consistency: changes/ dry / crumbly/ Egg white/ Not sure
Contraception method:	If Pill, have you had any problems taking Pill? Yes / No

Have you managed to conceive naturally before?	Yes	No
Miscarriage/Ectopic? Yes or No	**Details of weeks or number of miscarriages**	
Do you have any children? Yes or No	**Type of delivery?**	
Any sexually transmitted infections? **If yes, please circle.**	<u>You</u> Yes/ No PID / Chlamydia	<u>Partner</u> Yes / No STIs/Mumps
How long have you been trying for a baby?		
Any Investigations? Tube Patency etc Please tick box:	Tubal Clear □ Blockage □ Left □ Right □	
Treatment Cycles IVF/ICSI/FET/IUI. If yes, please state:		
Has your partner had a Semen Analysis performed? Yes / No **DNA Fragmentation? Yes / No** **Result? – please tick boxes**	Normal □ Low □ No sperm □ Comments on: Morphology □ Motility □ Viscosity □ Sluggish □	
Any other relevant medical history including recent surgery/gynae?		
Details of any supplements or medication:		
Can you take/tolerate Vitamin B Yes /No		

Client signature: _____   Date: _____

Therapist signature: _____   Date: _____

Body weight

Body weight can affect a client's fertility status. Being too heavy is as bad as being too light. Both ends of the spectrum can affect the function and regularity of the menstrual cycle by influencing hormone production, in particular oestrogen. More commonly, periods may be very scant, light, short and irregular, or they may be experienced as very heavy, clotty, long and infrequent or a mix of these. With these clients, I am encouraging them to look at their diet, keep a food diary, exercise and either reduce or try to add to their weight. For clients who are lighter in weight the addition of 6-8lbs can make a difference to the function and regularity of the cycle. For those who are heavier, the reduction of 10lbs plus can also affect an improvement of the cycle flow, differences to levels of pain experienced and general feelgood factors.

Emotional and physical conditions

Emotional and physical conditions will impact on how the body assimilates nutrition and how the body overall copes with these variables. What goes on in our mind is not separate from what goes on in our body. If the body is anxious and stressed, hormone levels will be affected. Indeed, all body systems will be affected to some degree and the immune system compromised. The female will be affected by overproduction of cortisol and a depletion of progesterone will occur, resulting in lowering of their fertility.

Those clients who exercise to extreme, the 'gym bunnies', will compromise their fertility. Those females who 'run the roads', who continually are running and undertaking heavy cardio exercising, will affect their hormone balance. Cortisol production, which is converted from the production of progesterone via the adrenals, will rise and progesterone will drop, as will their fertility and they will also see a rise in oestrogen and testosterone levels which may lead to erratic and irregular menstrual bleeds, or none at all. Cortisol is a beneficial hormone which is used as part of the 'fight or flight' response, but when it is placed under extreme pressure and is continually required, in the case of high impact exercise, it can derail your body's most important functions. It can also lead to a number of health problems, such as lower fertility or adrenal diseases, poor sleep or digestive issues.

Exercise is necessary but it should be much gentler and less taxing on the body systems. Walking, pilates, yoga are much more beneficial to the body as a whole. Sustained sympathetic nervous system dominance is detrimental to all body systems. The reproductive system is also strongly affected. There are clients who state that they can't give up their running and I try to suggest that they reduce the number of times they do this in the week, such as once weekly and perhaps take up some gentler forms of exercise. There are those who cannot make these changes, and as therapists, you may find that you will work with them much longer to see, for example, a change in their cycle.

Another important aspect of exercising is to do with the male partner. It is those males who consume protein shakes. There are those shakes which have been found to be detrimental to the life cycle of the sperm. They have been shown to decrease the quality and quantity of sperm. I tend to discourage any consumption of these drinks and suggest water instead. Good quality water is important to ensure function of the organs and systems. Hydrating the body will encourage fascia to slide and glide over body organs and prevent adhesions, which occur when fascia isn't well hydrated and is stuck, especially to areas such as bowel, where it could impinge on movement and peristaltic transit. Nutrition and water are integral to digestive function from the moment we eat food through to the act of defaecation. As Gillian McKeith says, 'we are what we eat'.

Bowel habit

I always ask about bowel habit as part of the initial consultation - remember I said that gut health is an important consideration. Bowel habit can vary enormously between clients and I'm sure as therapists, you will have clients confide in you about the regularity of their bowel habit, and through the use of reflexology you will feel a variety of imbalances such as congestion, firmness or popping when working the clients' intestines. Regular bowel movements are essential to good health and are an indicator to a healthy diet. If your client tells you that they do not go for many days, the stool can back up in the intestines and harden. It can also putrefy, releasing toxins. This can lead to autotoxication, as the toxins are absorbed across the wall of the colon into the bloodstream. The muscle tone of the colon wall is also weakened, so peristalsis weakens, leading to a sluggish bowel and further faeces transit problems. If this goes on for too long, it starts to pose a risk to the client's health and can damage their organs. Therefore, it is so important to health to ensure that the bowel functions regularly.

As reflexologists we are good at applying moves to support the intestines and encourage movement. Other ways clients can improve peristalsis in the gut is through increased fibre, water, movement, removing irritating foods such as spicy foods, or sugar sweeteners such as those that end in 'ol' - sorbitol, mannitol, and xylitol, fatty foods or alcohol or caffeinated drinks.

In the west, we probably have the most inefficient lavatories for defecation. They hold the anus too high, which means the angle of the rectum impedes the ejection of faeces. The best position is a squat, which corrects this angle and eases bowel evacuation. The easiest way to achieve this on a conventional toilet, is to place a few thick books or a shallow step under your feet as you sit and tuck your feet under your thighs as much as possible. Release will now be much easier. Remember, straining creates haemorrhoids.

Occupational stress

Occupational stress, which many of our clients experience, can cause imbalances on many levels: females may see the effects of this in the menstrual cycle – irregularity, consisting of spotting, short, light bleeds, long heavy clotty bleeds and all created by imbalanced hormones, such as progesterone and oestrogen. (This is discussed in greater detail above.) This will impact on their life in an emotional and physical way by creating dis-ease and as we reflexologists are aware, is seen so clearly in the feel of the feet and the reflexes. This is such an important topic, as not everyone can cope adequately with stress to keep their life and their fertility in equilibrium.

Stress can manifest in so many ways: insomnia, musculoskeletal discomfort/pain, inability to concentrate, diminished appetite or the need for comfort eating and thought congestion. Thoughts and emotions impinge greatly on how the female cycle works, affecting the levels of hormones, which in turn affect the optimum production of the menstrual cycle including ovulation, the bleed and ultimately the client's fertility.

The time when your client is wanting a child is generally the time when they are trying to establish their career, create a nurturing home environment and maintain their loving relationship. All these areas of your life demand time. There is a lot to juggle and cope with… and then you have menstrual cycles which may or may not be working properly…the client has come off the pill after x years…or they're now actively trying to get pregnant after not using any contraception …or their partner's having fertility issues such as erectile dysfunction or low sperm count or you're part of a same sex partnership and the obstacles you're having to face seem insurmountable and there's menstrual issues appearing here… and the stress is building!

As I have already said, stress can be experienced in so many ways as we are all individuals, and all have varying levels of coping mechanisms.

I'm always extremely keen to discover what my client's occupation is; remember this can take up the majority of their daily life. How the client manages their work-related stress will indicate their recognition of it and their ability to help themselves. Or does it require some input from us as reflexologists to steer them in the right direction? Remember this is all part of their day to day self-care.

Case study:

I recall a client who is self-employed, of slight stature, pale skin colouring overall and was adamant that she didn't have any problems with stress, when completing the consultation form. I visualised how she entered my treatment room that day, she was 10 minutes late, flustered, and rushed in through the door ready to jump on to the couch, without any thought of telling me anything about herself. On settling on to the chair she chatted, giving me an outline of her history and completed the consultation form. Most of her answers were two- or three-word replies; I had to ask her about her written responses on the form. It was difficult to tease more complex responses at this stage as she seemed guarded. I wondered if there was a more emotional level to this lady (I eventually discovered, as we came towards the end of the form, that she had previously had 3 miscarriages and had sought further support and guidance from Fertility/Gynae/ Obst consultants to no avail). She was protecting her emotional self deeply. This later showed up in her feet in the chest/lungs/ diaphragm, thyroid area, liver and gallbladder. Grieving, emotional anguish and anger remained and needed support. Through recommendation, another consultant was found, who could review her clinical notes and give her the answers she needed to help her move forward whilst I continued to support her using reflexology and other tools.

Another question on the form asked about her sleep pattern and she proudly declared that she had 7-8 hours' sleep daily and there was no problem with this. I've heard this so often and I thought inwardly that the feet will tell me whether any of these declarations are true. On touching the feet, they were inflexible, very stiff and cold. That's fine, as sometimes when new clients come, they are entering unfamiliar territory with an unfamiliar therapist, and the feet can reflect this apprehension, by being stiff and sometimes inflexible. The brain was as firm as a brick as I thumb walked it, as was the pineal. It took some time performing relaxation moves and deep breathing to achieve some flexibility and relaxation. I performed some work on the vagus nerve to help with relaxation, at both the start and the finish. At the end of the session, the feet had warmed up.

On further questioning and feedback, I told the client what I had found, and she laughed loudly and nervously. She admitted that she did have lots of chatter in her head, caused by lots of targets and deadlines she had to meet with work and that it could take an hour or more, for her to get to sleep, but once achieved she did sleep! We discussed several options that might aid her getting to sleep. She liked the idea of short 10-minute meditations, which she could use to help with the chatter and support her getting to sleep.

She was amazed that her feet could show so much. I told her which foot I could feel where she had lots of activity meaning that this is the side she was ovulating on and that I could feel a prominent follicle on this side (she texted me several days later to confirm that she attended for a transvaginal scan and the specialist had confirmed that she had a follicle on the same side). The scan confirmed what I could feel. With practice and developing sensitivity of fingers and thumbs, fertility reflexologists can feel follicles on the ovary.

Before she left my room, I gave her homework to do, which included working her ankles and her wrists. I also asked her to wear socks 24/7, which included in bed. She agreed to do this, as she felt her feet being so cold could possibly be another factor why she finds it so difficult to get to sleep. My rationale for the socks was to warm the reproductive reflexes and help with blood circulation. I also asked her to eat warming foods such as soups, stews, curries, and use foods such as ginger (use in teas or food) garlic and small amounts of chilli. I also asked the client to do deep breathing exercises, as they are good for activating the vagus nerve and helped with the feel-good factor too!

At her next visit her feet were much more pliable for working, still cool but the feet warmed up much quicker, which I recorded. Her brain and pineal showed a slight improvement; she hadn't looked at the short meditations which we had discussed, but rather she had started to take an evening walk with her partner. So even though she didn't do what we agreed, she did find a way of relaxing in nature and she shared it in the company of her partner. The learning here is identifying the imbalance and offering ways of supporting it in a way which interests the client, or by sowing the seed and letting the client find the way that fits their lifestyle – as long as it happens, it's ok.

She had ordered supplements for both herself and her husband, which arrived the day before the second session and both had started these. They both had discussed their diets and although they were good, with freshly made foods and fruit, they decided to make a concerted effort to stay focussed and increase their water intake, which wasn't great, and eat more fruit (berries) as snacks. They both work from home and were great coffee advocates, and the effort was in replacing some cups of coffee with water or herbal teas!

Quietening the head wasn't the only issue this client had, but sometimes you need to start at the beginning, supporting for example sleep issues, which will impact and improve other areas of fertility. One important aspect pertaining to this is melatonin and the sleep/wake cycle. The role of this hormone is diverse, such as aiding the body's antioxidant defences and helping to regulate blood pressure, body temperature and cortisol levels, as well as sexual and immune function. The production of melatonin is at its greatest while we are asleep and can help provide 7-8 hours of quality sleep. Poor or broken sleep patterns caused by using devices such as laptops and smartphones before bedtime can have a negative impact on melatonin secretion, circadian rhythms and sleep. This recurrent disturbed sleep can affect levels of the hormone and this can adversely influence levels of oestrogen in the female body, which will affect fertility (and other hormones such as progesterone levels) and the menstrual cycle.

So it is important to correlate this information to what the client has relayed to you, about the pattern of their menstrual cycle and their bleed. What you are trying to do is build up an interconnecting picture with the information being provided and extrapolating gaps in what you have been told, based on the evidence on the feet and physical presentation. Sometimes, you need to be a detective. I suggest to clients that they should be turning off devices by 9pm at night and not taking them into the bedroom to avoid upsetting the body's circadian rhythms.

This client's cycle ranged between 25 – 28 days and began with brown coloured spotting followed by bright red bleed, with no pain prior to the onset, or during the bleed, rather slight cramping at day 2, nil else. Usually the bleed could last between 3-5 days. At 3 days it was quite short. The client was aware of her ovulation day, as she experienced ovulatory pain. She stated that she ovulated at day 16, which for a 25 day cycle is quite late, when you consider the length of the luteal phase. Calculating day 16 for ovulation, 3-4 days for bleed provides 8 days for a luteal phase, which is short in length and could be an indicator for miscarriages. As this client has had 3 miscarriages in the past, I considered this as a possibility. Fertility doctors don't look at the detail of the cycle and make such deductions; they are looking for a more obvious cause such as a genetic deficiency, or the failure of cell division within the embryo. I consider that a significant oversight on their part.

The luteal phase is the final phase of the menstrual cycle and lasts from the day of ovulation to the last day before the next period. The luteal phase is named after the corpus luteum – a structure that grows in the ovary. It is dominated by progesterone, which is the hormone responsible for the rise in the Basal Body Temperature (BBT). If progesterone is low, temperature could show as low on chart, or there could be low levels of T3, which we can assess for an imbalance by working the thyroid and thyroid helper. The luteal phase is considered to be short if it lasts less than 10 days. A short luteal phase doesn't give the uterine lining a chance to grow and develop enough to support implantation of a growing baby. As a result, it can be harder to get pregnant, or it might take you longer to conceive. Or it may mean, if the client does get pregnant that the progesterone level drops early, and the pregnancy can't be sustained.

On the other hand, a long luteal phase may be due to a hormone imbalance like polycystic ovary syndrome (PCOS). How can we as therapists support this defect? I recommend using the stimulation techniques for the Luteal Phase Defect (LPD) in weekly sessions, and the client completing her homework. I also suggest additional B6 which can be used to extend this part of the menstrual cycle alongside using reflexology.

Her smear history showed that her smear was up to date and results were normal. There was no history of abnormal smears or colposcopy treatment. I asked the client if there was any difficulty obtaining the smear and she stated that she was required to place her hands under her gluteals to prop herself for the nurse to get a view of the cervix – this can be an indication that the uterus is tilted (meaning that your uterus is naturally tilted toward your spine, not your belly button). In such a presentation, the suggested position for effective intercourse would be 'doggy style' (on your hands and knees, with penetration from behind) as the best way for the sperm to reach their destination, and as it usually takes about 15 minutes for sperm to reach the cervix, the client can lie back and relax for that length of time before getting up.

From a reflexology stance I'm also thinking that it would be beneficial to assess the psoas muscle, as tightness of this muscle could also impinge on the pelvis. Such tightness can be the result of some forms of gym exercise. As well as working the psoas I will assess the spinal innervation thoracic 12 (T12).

Furthermore, many types of lubricants, and even saliva, can slow sperms' motility and speed; it's best to skip them when trying to conceive. If a client tells me she's using lubrication I'm wondering if there is a problem with arousal, or does she suffer from poor natural lubrication of her mucosal membranes, especially cervical mucus – that's how intimate, we need to get here! I'll ask her about her eyes – gritty or dry eyes, or dry lips or mouth. If this appears to be a problem, I'm thinking that there's a deficiency in Omega 7 (Palmitoleic Acid). If there is poor lubrication of these areas, it's probable that cervical mucus may be low. I show clients a chart made up of images of the sequential changes the mucus goes through during the normal cycle (there's also a copy in their booklet). It shows clients the changes of colour and consistency of mucus throughout the cycle and I ask them if they notice these changes taking place. Some clients will have a good understanding of how their body works, whilst others have never paid attention to this process. Some even display disgust at the thought of examining their cervical mucus. It is a learning curve for many as they progress on this journey.

Ways to counteract this deficiency are to increase good fats such as avocado oil intake, Macadamia nuts or oil, or Sea Buckthorn Oil capsules (my preferred option) or Evening Primrose Oil - EPO (however, those clients with cystic breasts should not use this supplement). Clients can choose to supplement or not supplement, to enhance cervical mucus and/or use reflexology instead which I have found has supported many of my clients with limited cervical mucus, to observe increased cervical mucus, along with noting the changes occurring throughout the cycle. Those clients who chose to supplement with EPO, particularly those who have poor cervical mucus with little change to consistency being noted, are asked to take this daily for 3 months in the first instance, as it usually takes this length of time to see a significant change to the mucus. If a change is observed sooner – that is that the mucus goes through all the consistency changes seen in normal mucus within 3 months - then the client should adjust EPO to take it from the first day of the cycle to the day of ovulation, then stopping until day 1 of the following cycle up to ovulation and so on for a further 3 cycles at least. Some clients try to wean themselves off the EPO thereafter, whilst other prefer to continue.

Cervical mucus

So far, we have discussed the ways of increasing cervical mucus, but what we must also consider is that there are occasions when cervical mucus will diminish in females, who have never had a problem with its production. This can happen when spring allergies or forms of rhinitis arrive as the weather gets warmer. GPs will prescribe an antihistamine, the role of which is to dry up secretions, and it isn't selective in the secretions that are reduced. So, it is always beneficial to be aware of this problem occurring. There are numerous homeopathic and herbal remedies that can be used as an alternative for this purpose.

As reflexologists, cervical mucus is an important tool for us to note the changes happening for the client – therefore it is important that the client feeds this information to the therapist at each visit. As it changes throughout the cycle, it informs the therapist that the cycle is functioning as it should, or it may highlight that there is an issue with the cycle and hormones. Changes in mucus normally goes from thick/opaque/tacky, to creamy, to slippery/clear/stretchy, or even watery. Throughout most of the cycle, the cervical mucus is fairly acidic and hostile toward sperm. But in the days leading up to ovulation, the acidity of cervical mucus decreases becoming more alkaline, to allow sperm to travel and support sperm nutrition.

Any clients identified with poor mucus through questioning, I will demonstrate the techniques to, and they are instructed to perform these at home daily. The techniques involve stimulating the ovary on the lateral aspect of the ankle and stimulating the uterus on the medial aspect. These moves can be performed together on each foot. I recommend that these moves are done 3-4 times daily, with pressure and I show the client the pressure to apply for at least one minute, by working on the client's feet. I also like them to stimulate the same reflexes on the wrists for the same amount of time (wrists are usually easier to do when at work as it's less obvious), whilst ankles can be done at home – breakfast, evening and before bed.

If these tasks are completed daily as requested, the client will see a very quick response to increased cervical mucus – I mean it can happen within days and depends where the client is in their cycle, as to how quickly the client will see this change occur. Please note when demonstrating these techniques to clients, I don't highlight where either reflex is found on the feet as I don't want the client getting hung up on whether they are working the reflex either correctly, or in the correct area. I ask them to visualise a line from the back of the ankle, running below the malleolus and finishing at the cuboid notch/tuberosity on the lateral side and mirror this on the medial side, and state that they need to work this entire area, using fingers or thumb. I think it is easier if they work both sides together.

Another suggestion I make to clients is to get their partner to do this for them and they can do the same moves on their other half's feet – it's a good move for males with poor sperm results – this will be discussed in more detail later.

When the client approaches ovulation, there will be other symptoms or changes such as: sexual desire, breast tenderness, maintained Basal Body Temperature increase, bloating, hormonal headaches and PMS. These are very individual and not all clients will experience all or many of these symptoms, at the time of ovulation. Some clients will use other means of forecasting ovulation, such as an Ovulation Predicator Kit (OPK personally, I do not recommend these as I find them inaccurate) or the OvuSense monitor, that the client inserts into the vagina to record their temperature. It states that it will alert you up to **24-hours before you ovulate**, based on your in-cycle data.

My question is WHY? Why would clients insert a device which uses an Electro Magnetic Field (EMF) to provide them with the information to alert them when they are reaching ovulation, WHEN as reflexologists, we are trying to encourage our clients to use more NATURAL methods to achieve a pregnancy such as observing mucus change, record temperature using a thermometer, eat clean, fresh food, drink plenty of clean water, reduce processed foods and perform gentle exercise etc. This, to me, goes against the whole ethos of what we are trying to achieve.

Numerous clients have admitted that they used this monitor prior to coming to see me, and found it expensive and not very reliable in its forecast, which increased emotional upset and sometimes it created more hormonal upset than had been experienced prior to starting with the device. Quite a few clients commented when nothing happened each month i.e. pregnancy, this added to their stress level.

It is much better to encourage your client to take responsibility for their health and become involved in what happens within. However, adding to a client's chemical load is wrong and damaging in the long run as there is not adequate research performed on these devices, to know the long-term side-effects on the female body. There is more than enough EMF outside of the body without adding to the internal environment whilst on this journey.

Sperm quality

Other forms of EMF can be received from the mobile phone. We cannot survive without our mobile phones. Yet research has shown them to negatively impact sperm quality. Researchers at Cleveland Clinic have shown that the use of mobile phones decreases sperm count, viability and morphology. The longer a phone is kept in a hip pocket, the more damage can be inflicted. It is thought to be a combination of heat from the mobile through the emission of radiofrequency and oxidative stress.

Researchers have stated for a long time that heat impairs the quality of sperm, which is why the male body was designed in such a way, that the scrotal sack remains outside the body at a lower temperature than the remainder of the body.

The production of sperm – spermatogenesis- occurs in the seminiferous tubules that form the bulk of each testis. The process begins at puberty, after which time sperm are produced constantly throughout a man's life. One production cycle, from spermatogonia through to formed sperm, takes approximately 72 days.

A new cycle starts approximately every 16 days, although this timing is not synchronous across the seminiferous tubules. Sperm counts - the total number of sperm a man produces - slowly decline after age 35, and some studies suggest that smoking can lower sperm counts irrespective of age.

Sperm are smaller than most cells in the body; in fact, the volume of a sperm cell is 85,000 times less than that of the female egg. Approximately 100 to 300 million sperm are produced each day, whereas women typically ovulate only one oocyte (egg) per month.

The structure of sperm cells has 3 sections, namely the head, mid-piece, and tail region. The head of the sperm contains the extremely compact haploid nucleus with very little cytoplasm.

A structure called the acrosome covers most of the head of the sperm cell as a "cap" that is filled with lysosomal enzymes important for preparing sperm to participate in fertilization.

Tightly packed mitochondria fill the mid-piece of the sperm. ATP produced by these mitochondria will power the flagellum, which extends from the neck and the mid-piece through the tail of the sperm, enabling it to move the entire sperm cell. The central strand of the flagellum, the axial filament, is formed from one centriole inside the maturing sperm cell during the final stages of spermatogenesis.

Sperm make up only 5 percent of the final volume of semen, the thick, milky fluid that the male ejaculates.

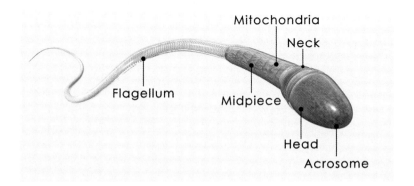

Increasing sperm count

Here are a few of the more natural techniques and treatments that have been shown to be effective at increasing sperm count. Studies have shown improvements in as little as 1 month, with maximum benefit often seen after about 3 months of regular cooling (e.g. icing down your testicles once a day).

Testicular cooling: intentionally cooling the testicle using an ice pack placed in the underwear has been shown to be an effective way to increase sperm count. It is recommended that men avoid hot baths, tight underwear, replacing these with loose boxer shorts, sitting with laptops on their laps, stopping the use of heated car seats, or sitting in hot tubs for periods of time.

When we consider that it takes several months to produce good quality sperm these suggestions are something that males could adopt, coupled with dietary changes including supplementation for 2-3 months before they see a change in sperm results.

Several studies have endorsed improvements in sperm count in as little as two months, with the use of male fertility supplement blends.

Supplementation should include an all-round male fertility multi-vitamin, Co-enzyme Q10, in the form of Ubiquinol to aid reduction of DNA damage in sperm, improve motility, count and morphology: Fish oil – cold pressed and L-Carnitine (this may be present in multi-vitamin but generally not in the dose required for optimum daily intake. Reduce alcohol consumption, smoking, red meat, reduce sugary foods and increased brightly coloured foods and oily fish.

Weight loss: many studies have shown that being overweight inhibits sperm production. Only a few studies have looked at changes in sperm count over time, as men lose weight in order to increase sperm count, but those studies are very encouraging. For example, a 2011 Danish study showed that during a 14-week weight loss program, the men who lost the most weight showed the highest improvement in sperm count.

Exercise: regular exercise goes hand in hand with weight loss and overall fitness. A recent study showed that men who go jogging several times a week improved their sperm count meaningfully in about 6 months. Those males who become 'mamils' (middle-aged men in lycra) and cycle around the country in their tight fitting lycra attire add significantly to their fertility issues, due to increased temperature around scrotal area and the seating position on the bicycle.

The male partner who has a semen analysis (SA) result of low sperm count, or sluggish sperm, can also reduce abnormal forms and can possibly see changes in SA results after 3-4 months or up to 6 months, if they implement dietary and lifestyle changes which include the use of fertility supplements such as IMPRYL or Proxeed Plus for men. Both products are designed to improve low sperm count, sluggish sperm or abnormal forms, alongside 12 sessions of once weekly reflexology using the stimulation techniques I apply to the females.

The techniques are used primarily to stimulate the male reproductive reflexes to aid sperm production. Male clients should continue with the same homework moves as discussed for the female client for at least 12 weeks, which should culminate in a repeat SA to assess any improvements.

I try to get clients to embrace all the recommendations I make for changes in their lifestyle: dietary, supplementation and stress management, alongside the use of reflexology and, as necessary, fertility massage and their homework tasks. I am keen for clients to view this experience as a two-way journey and I encourage them to become involved, as I can't fix them alone. They must play their part and thereby demonstrate their commitment to the journey.

The client's role

The client's role includes the changes suggested, the homework tasks, supplementation and any other observations requested of them, such as cervical mucus or temperature recording. I must admit, some clients do not like to record this, as they feel it adds another level of stress to perform this daily. If this is the case, I don't force this, as I would rather prevent more blockages than add to them. It may be an area a client will undertake as they progress through the sessions.

Temperature

It's amazing the difference we see between our clients, as others have begun to monitor their temperature when they first attend and can provide you with an array of information for consideration. Usually clients have an App on their Smart phone which they can share. I particularly like 'Fertility Friend' as an App. It's been around longer than some of the others and it is very supportive, sending you lots of emails and advice, whilst there is a multitude of ovulation trackers available. It has a gallery of graphs to help with reading recordings.

If clients are going to record their temperature, they require a digital thermometer solely for this use. They need to decide if they are going to take their temperature under their tongue or the axilla (armpit) and always use the designated area. The client must take the temperature each morning at the same time and before they put their feet out of bed otherwise this will change the body's core temperature, which is what the client is attempting to read and record.

Note the temperature, and when convenient record it on the Fertility App. This in turn will provide a record of what is happening with the cycle during the month. Most Apps can forecast once you have provided your menstrual history at start-up of the App, showing when the client possibly will be ovulating. Of course, the forecast is only as good as the information that the client is feeding in. The client can input information about headaches, a cold, other bodily upsets, PMS etc and when they are having intercourse, or what the quality of their cervical mucus is like. So, lots of valuable information can be stored and related to the monthly cycle.

I am interested to see if the graph shows if the cycle looks normal and what the temperature range looks like. Does it show an ovulatory spike and how the temperature is expressed at the second part of the cycle, the length of the Luteal Phase, to assess if it functions properly, or is there a defect present more commonly known as the Luteal Phase defect?

I'm thinking if the temperature drops below 35.8 that there could be a subclinical issue with the thyroid, even though clients may have had their bloods done and I have scrutinized them and they fall within the normal range (clients are asked for copies of their blood results and semen analysis). The important assessment is what the feet show on the thyroid reflex.

Reflexology

Remember, we as reflexologists regard the thyroid as the third ovary and I'm keen to link these areas together, observing and feeling what is happening during this time from my perspective, and also what, if anything, the client is feeling, such as lethargy, and I will note this in their notes.

The repetition of continuing to encourage clients to feed back at each session about cervical mucus or any other experiences, will provide you the therapist, with the specific symptoms or changes happening for this client, and you can monitor these and observe what is happening in relation to the recommended techniques used at the stage of the client's cycle.

Note what visible responses you as the therapist are feeling or seeing on the feet, as well as what the client feels during this also. The feedback that the client provides at each visit requires you as the therapist to record detailed notes, as you learn the intricacies of each client.

I have noted that some clients mention that they feel as if their ovaries and uterus begin to feel more energised once they start to do their exercises, and there are times during each reflexology session, I have observed very noticeable responses from feet, toes or legs, or the client reports the experiences they are feeling in the knees, legs or thigh areas when applying the various techniques used for stimulation. This tells me that energy is moving, and communication of the various meridians and nervous and fascial pathways are taking place, which is all positive.

For those clients from whom I don't receive as much responsive feedback, I'm always concerned that they are not performing their homework. I always check this at each visit and try to encourage compliance. If the client is struggling to complete what is asked, I will always do more work to the reproductive areas, stimulate the hypothalamus and pituitary several times during the session, and reassess links several times to monitor responses.

Perform lots of relaxation to ensure the client is completely chilled before the session is completed. For these clients it will take more sessions to achieve the responses I am trying to achieve, with the reproductives and endocrines. I find the clients who do everything requested of them get much quicker responses and regulation of the cycle and temperature (if recording), than those who don't.

Interestingly, those clients whose temperature is 35.8 and below, if they do their homework, take supplementation, improve their diets etc usually will see a fairly quick improvement of their temperature, than those who just make a half-hearted attempt and it is easy to identify those from their recordings.

Changes during the cycle

So, let us consider the changes which happen during the cycle:

- During the **follicular phase**: the body starts to produce more oestrogen which peaks at ovulation, whilst progesterone has remained low. During the latter part of week 2, testosterone starts to rise. When this happens, it tends to make the female more impulsive, daring and competitive. Libido is high during week 2, however, when testosterone spikes, it boosts the libido even higher. When the day of ovulation is reached this marks the start of the Luteal Phase, progesterone begins to rise rapidly, whereas oestrogen is dropping, although at the end of week 3 it rises again before dropping. During this phase the appetite can increase under the influence of progesterone as preparation for the body to eat for 2. It's in case a pregnancy happens.

How does **cervical mucus** appear in consistency and texture during the menstrual cycle?

- **During your menstrual period**. Blood will cover the mucus, so not as obvious during these days.

- **After period**. Immediately following your period, there may be a few dry days. On these days, clients may not notice any discharge.

- **Before ovulation**. Now the body produces more viscous mucus before an egg is released, or before ovulation occurs. It may be yellow, white, or cloudy. The mucus may feel gluey or stretchy in consistency.

- **Immediately before ovulation**. Just prior to ovulation, your oestrogen levels are rising. You may see more clear, stretchy, watery and slippery mucus. This mucus may remind you of the consistency of egg whites.

- **During ovulation**. The clear, stretchy mucus that is the consistency of egg whites will be present during ovulation. The texture and pH of this mucus are protective for sperm. For this reason, if you are trying to conceive, have sex before ovulating. If clients are recording their temperature and/or observing cervical mucus, this should help them identify their fertile window. It is better to have baby dancing (intercourse) the day prior to ovulation to ensure that the sperm are ready to greet the egg, rather than have sperm chasing the egg on the day of ovulation. At ovulation, the cervix opens slightly to enable sperm to pass through. It is a difficult and challenging terrain for the sperm. Watch the youTube video **https://www.youtube.com/ watch?v=_5OvgQW6FG4**

The wet and viscous mucus also serves as the vehicle to transport sperm to the cervix, as well as provide nutrition to the sperm, providing energy to keep them active as they wait on the arrival of the ripe egg.

The lifespan of the sperm is longer than that of the egg (ova). Generally, the sperm can live for 2–5 days, whilst the egg is around 12–24 hours (I usually err on the side of caution with eggs and say 12 hrs, as it depends on individual genetics and client health etc). If a client recognises or experiences Mittelschmerz Pain (ovulation pain) and can pin-point this to a time eg. 7am, they haven't had intercourse in the last few days and think 'tonight's the night', by the time they get home from work and intercourse takes place after 9pm for example, the couple will have possibly missed the opportunity of fertilisation taking place, as the egg quality will have deteriorated if the egg lifespan is 12 hours.

■ **After ovulation**. There will be less discharge after ovulation. It may turn thicker, cloudy, or gluey in appearance and texture. The purpose is to now keep sperm out. Some women experience dry days during this time, as the cervix closes.

The client I discussed earlier has mentioned that she spots the first day of her bleed. When clients talk about spotting, at this part of the bleed, I disregard this as being the first day of the cycle. This spotting usually is an indication of old, retained blood from the previous cycle, which has not come away, which is why it is darker in colour.

Day 1 is the day when the client has a true red bleed. The client admitted that she counted the day of spotting as day 1, where in fact day 2 has become day 1 as it is the day when the client has a bright red bleed. This means the length of the cycle bleed has changed and the client stated she had 3 days to the cycle, it is now reduced to 2 days (2 days is short) – or if it lasts for 5 days it is reduced to 4 days.

Depending on the information the client has shared about the colour, length, consistency and pain I'm starting to build a picture of what is happening to the hormones: oestrogen and progesterone specifically. If these hormones are not in balance during the cycle, it means that one or other will not be functioning during either the follicular or the luteal phase of the cycle, and this will have numerous implications for the client's fertility. If the hormones are out of balance, each of the hormones will be affected. This means if one is low, the other will be high.

When you understand how the menstrual cycle works and the hormones involved in each phase, you can begin to recognise which hormone/s are not functioning properly and recognise client's symptoms when they mention this, and this helps you put the pieces of the jigsaw together. This all takes time, practice and experience when dealing with your clients, so don't be hard on yourself if you don't seem to grasp it all in one go. Remember, Rome wasn't built in a day and neither will your client's jigsaw. It may take weeks to piece it altogether, as you and your client bond and build up communication. There will be those clients whom you meet who are very in tune with their bodies and there will be those who are not. Your role will be as educator, to help them understand their cycle and observe and listen to their bodies.

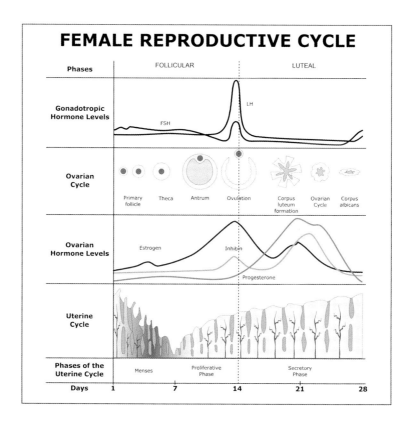

FEMALE REPRODUCTIVE CYCLE

*I have commented that 3 days is short – relate these 3 days to the function of oestrogen and this helps with our understanding. Oestrogen's main function during the cycle, following ovulation, is to create the lining of the uterus for the implantation of the blastocyst (fertilised egg). The endometrium grows to a thick, blood vessel-rich, glandular tissue layer which will support this. If the level of oestrogen is too low the lining will be too thin to allow implantation to take place and the blastocyst will not be able to implant and the pregnancy will not continue.

The purpose of oestrogen

- controls the growth of the uterine lining during the menstrual cycle and at the beginning of a pregnancy
- causes breast changes in teenagers and women who are pregnant
- is involved in bone and cholesterol metabolism
- regulates food intake, body weight, glucose metabolism, and insulin sensitivity-particularly relevant with PCOS clients.

Low oestrogen can lead to:

- Headaches
- Flashes
- Night sweats and vaginal dryness
- Inability to ovulate
- Thin uterine lining

High oestrogen can lead to:

- Heavy clotty bleeds
- Causing the body to manufacture stress hormone cortisol
- Poor sleep due to reduction in melatonin

The purpose of progesterone

- It has important roles in the menstrual cycle and in early stages of pregnancy.
- Works with oestrogen to release a mature egg.
- After ovulation the corpus luteum releases progesterone until the mature placenta takes over.
- Encourages lining to become sticky and enable implantation of the fertilised egg to occur.
- This in turn stimulates the placenta into growth and helps maintain a lower level of progesterone throughout the pregnancy.

- Inhibits muscular contractions of the uterus that would probably cause the wall to reject the adhering egg.
- During implantation and gestation, progesterone appears to decrease the maternal immune response to allow for the acceptance of the pregnancy.

Low progesterone can lead to:
- Inability to produce egg at ovulation
- Infertility or miscarriages
- Uterine bleeding or irregular periods and spotting

High Progesterone can lead to:
- Stomach upset
- Change of appetite
- Weight gain
- Acne
- High likelihood of twin pregnancy

Outwardly, what the client reports about her bleed, is the number of days, the colour and consistency and any other symptoms experienced. Thus, a thin lining results in a short, light bleed.

A thin endometrium can also be a sign of decreased fertility in general. Poor ovarian response is associated with a thin endometrium – this may or may not be age related. Young women can have a poor ovarian response, or poor egg quality, as well as older women – some older women can have a good ovarian response and egg quality – it can all be down to genetics or the quality of nutrition!

Also, important to note, repeated use of the fertility drug Clomid is known to negatively impact endometrial thickness, as it works on the hormone oestrogen.

To ensure implantation happens, the lining must achieve a depth (7mm - 8mm on average) which allows the blastocyst to bury into the endometrium and ensures the developing placenta will begin to secrete human chorionic gonadotropic hormone (hCG). This pregnancy hormone then signals the corpus luteum (on the ovaries) to keep producing progesterone, which maintains the endometrium during the first 12 weeks of pregnancy, until the mature placenta takes over the role of maintaining the pregnancy. Clients who continue to measure their temperature will note that their temperature remains high.

However, if the embryo doesn't implant into the endometrium, the corpus luteum will begin to break down, leading to decreasing levels of the hormone progesterone. When progesterone drops, the glands of the endometrium will stop secreting the fluids that were maintaining it. Also, with the withdrawal of progesterone, the spiral arteries that were supplying the endometrium with blood flow begin to constrict and the core body temperature begins to drop. This results in the breakdown of the endometrium. Finally, the endometrium is expelled from the uterus via menstruation, and the cycle begins again.

Balancing hormones – non ovulation

There are herbs which can be used, such as Agnus Castus, to balance the hormones oestrogen and progesterone. There is a tincture preparation which can be used for this purpose, although the company which produces this has been awarded a short licence from MHRA, which doesn't allow them to state this hormonal function on the Patient information Leaflet (PIL), as fertility is regarded as a long process and is therefore not covered by the licence.

I use this preparation with some clients (but not those with PCOS or Endometriosis) along with reflexology techniques. For PCOS clients, I encourage them to use a product consisting of Myo-inositol which regulates a number of hormones such as thyroid-stimulating hormone, follicle-stimulating hormone (FSH) and insulin.

For those who are not trained to use such products, I recommend reflexology for stimulating the reproductive reflexes and the endocrines – especially the hypothalamus and pituitary together, adrenals, thyroid alongside the uterus and ovary. I have a combination of techniques designed to be used for reproductive reflexes and endocrines, to influence a response and create communication and energy flow to support the cycle into normal function, to create harmony and balance.

I recommend weekly sessions generally. There are those clients, who are overweight, who have had a long timespan without a bleed and I suggest twice weekly sessions for the first 3-4 weeks to enhance the cycle, in conjunction with the client performing the homework techniques as previously pictured and discussed. I will reassess the outcomes following the first bleed after the use of these methods.

Questioning of the client will consist of wanting to know how the bleed started i.e. spotting or proper red bleed, the colour, length and was there any pain experienced, as well as how the client felt prior to the bleed starting.

The application of this approach, (seeing twice weekly for 3-4 weeks) appears to have a shock effect on the body, by making the body produce a bleed, usually between 4-6 weeks later. The second bleed can take much longer and requires patience and perseverance by both the client and the therapist. I explain this to the client at the first visit and, thereafter, I remind them of this. Once the third cycle has arrived it's usually a good sign that the cycle is starting to settle into a regular regime. However, it is not a sign to stop having regular reflexology, or forget about performing homework, as this can result in the cycle going back to its former routine.

The client needs to continue having their hormones stimulated, both by the therapist and themselves. If at this stage the client is unable to maintain weekly sessions, they must continue to do their homework daily in between reflexology attendances. If taking supplements, clients must maintain this routine too, as well as dietary habits.

The above approach can be used with those clients who don't ovulate (amenorrhea), those with PCOS, endometriosis, irregular periods and some of the unexplained fertility clients, depending on the history elicited concerning their bleed and cervical mucus. Again, weekly sessions using stimulation techniques, assessing the responses both visibly and by acknowledging how the energy is felt by the client and the therapist – is it buzzing, is it quiet or is there heat felt on any of the reflexes or via the techniques and what changes are observed with the cervical mucus.

Balancing hormones – ovulation

Clients who have regular periods and have been trying for a second or third pregnancy to no avail, even though they got pregnant without any bother before now, have what's referred to as 'secondary fertility' (the inability to become pregnant or to carry a baby to term, after previously giving birth). They have been struggling for 6 months or maybe a couple of years by the time they seek support. With these clients I will look at dietary habits, lifestyle factors including exercise, supplements, and stress levels, as any one of these may play a part.

Find out what the client knows about their cervical mucus; can they identify ovulation and when they think the important time for intercourse is, and what their normal bleed is like and what the cycle length is like. All these questions are on the consultation form. These clients don't usually have blood results to hand, as might those clients with primary fertility, and it's useful for them to get a hormone profile performed, which must also include the progesterone level. Hospital laboratories don't automatically perform the progesterone level as part of the hormones profile, as this is an expensive test. Therefore, I ask clients to make sure they request this test specifically.

Once these tests are performed and results go back to the GP, clients can get a copy, which they can share with the therapist.

Result ranges are clearly stated on each result and with practice, therapists can identify what is normal/abnormal. I provide examples and discuss, during my CPD course. Sometimes it's a matter of activating the hormones with this client. With the client, I go through all aspects of the consultation covering lifestyle, dietary habits etc and recommendations made. We then look at the practical approach, determined by the menstrual history and cycle. If it appears straightforward - regular menses, bright red bleeding from start, cervical mucus etc. - I will start by using both pre- and post-ovulation techniques, coupled with the stimulation of the hypothalamus and pituitary.

All of these techniques are dependent on where the client is in their menstrual cycle. I will follow this regime of moves until the client has achieved a further bleed, with routine changes noted in the cervical mucus up to ovulation and the length of the luteal phase, accompanied by temperature recording throughout. I continue seeing this client for 12 weekly sessions or more, depending on how the cycle is working. I may, at week 12 re-assessment if everything seems established, move to fortnightly. Then again there are those clients who prefer to maintain weekly sessions throughout and I will facilitate this. Clients can feel so many benefits of this approach – improvement in cycle regularity, in cycle bleed, less pain, length of cycle, reduction in hormonal headaches and feel good factors, such as relaxation and less stress.

Sometimes the client, although they appear to have a regular menstrual cycle with hormone function, as observed through production/consistency/texture changes of the cervical mucus, can't achieve a pregnancy. It could be semen quality which is the issue, or it may be egg quality. I'm making a very generalised statement here, as it's not always older clients who have poor egg quality. It can be younger women and, unless clients have their AMH/antral count performed, they will not be aware of this problem. GPs can't perform these tests; they need to be performed by a Fertility Specialist.

The AMH level for the Anti Mullerian Hormone, indicates the female's ability to produce eggs that can be fertilized for pregnancy. A woman's ovaries can produce thousands of eggs during her childbearing years. The number declines as a woman gets older. AMH levels help show how many potential egg cells a woman has left. This is known as the ovarian reserve. If a woman's ovarian reserve is high, she may have a better chance of getting pregnant. If the ovarian reserve is low, chances are the woman will have trouble getting pregnant.

Antral follicles are small follicles (about 2-9 mm in diameter) that can be seen, measured and counted with a transvaginal ultrasound. Antral follicles are also referred to as resting follicles. Antral follicle counts (along with female age) are by far the best tool that the medical field currently have for estimating ovarian reserve, the expected response to ovarian stimulating drugs, and the chance for successful pregnancy with in vitro fertilization. The number of antral follicles visible on ultrasound is indicative of the number of microscopic primordial follicles remaining in the ovary. Each primordial follicle contains an immature egg that can potentially develop and ovulate in the future.

This is the point at which the female can influence the quality of the developing mature egg, through the consumption of high-quality foods and supplements. Supplements such as Coenzyme Q10 (CoQ10), which helps with energy within the cell via the mitochondria of the cell. It also protects cells from oxidative damage. As you age, CoQ10 production slows, making the body less effective at protecting eggs from oxidative damage. Supplementing with CoQ10 seems to help and may even reverse this age-related decline in egg quality and quantity. Statins severely reduce CoQ10 levels.

Similarly, male sperm is susceptible to the effects of oxidative damage, which may result in reduced sperm count, poor sperm quality and infertility. Ubiquinol accounts for 90% of the CoQ10 in the blood and is the most absorbable form for client supplementation. Several studies have concluded that supplementing with CoQ10 may improve sperm quality, activity and concentration by increasing antioxidant protection. There's ongoing discussion that DHEA can be beneficial for females with diminished ovarian reserve, and several of the fertility clinics are making this recommendation.

Even so, it remains controversial, although there are studies which suggest that it improves egg numbers and quality. It may also reduce miscarriage risk by increasing the availability of chromosomally normal eggs, for those clients with poor egg reserve/quality. A concern which clients need to be aware of, is that it is a hormone and it may interfere with other medication and it isn't recommended for those with PCOS or those with a history of a hormone sensitive cancer. Other side effects are that it can result in severe acne, hair loss or facial hair in some women among other conditions. Therefore, clients need to be aware of this before considering use.

DHEA is a hormone precursor produced in the adrenals and ovaries and is critical for early ovarian follicle development, alongside testosterone, which aids this production in the female, so it's clear why it appears as an attractive option. Some have argued for testosterone supplementation in preference, but it has been shown that not all females can metabolise this well, compared to DHEA. One fertility specialist, Dr N Gleicher sees it as revolutionising fertility management in older females, or younger females with ovaries that have aged prematurely. There are several articles written, which show that women in their mid to late thirties have taken this hormone for 3-4 months and have achieved a pregnancy naturally, avoiding the need for IVF. If it's something that a client is interested in, it would be useful to get their level of DHEA-S and testosterone tested beforehand.

Verisana Laboratory can provide testing for DHEA and **Testosterone, as well as other hormone tests, gut tests etc**. **www.verisana.co.uk** and are based in Germany; it is a very friendly and helpful company.

The results of such tests can be discussed with a GP or a Naturopath. This hormone is made from cholesterol by the adrenal glands so foods that are rich in a variety of healthy fats such as coconut milk, organic butter, flax, avocados, olive oil, nuts, seeds, and purified cold pressed omega-3 fish oil supplements. Healthy protein sources to boost DHEA production include wild-caught fish, grass-fed red meat and free-range chicken, turkey, and eggs, can provide the body with the raw materials it needs to produce the hormone.

Vitamin D plays a particularly important role in healthy DHEA levels. I recommend getting regular sun exposure and/or supplementation (using vitamin D3) to maintain vitamin D levels.

Blocked fallopian tubes

Throughout, I have mentioned many of the various common conditions seen; another can be blocked fallopian tube(s), ovarian cysts or fibroids. Again, depending on the menstrual history and all the components of this gleaned from the client, I recommend SerraPlus (derived from the silkworm) which is a natural chelation/anti-inflammatory proteolytic enzyme, which digests tissue causing blockages, adhesions, benign tumours or cysts. This enzyme, used in combination with weekly reflexology techniques, supplementation and a nutritious diet, can dissolve, resolve or reduce such conditions.

Sometimes in conjunction with reflexology for conditions such as cysts or fibroids, I will also recommend the client use castor oil packs. These can be used in the comfort of the client's home following an instruction leaflet, which I supply. They too, are beneficial and should be used for 3 months in the first instance, using cold pressed castor oil and red flannel as a wrap.

Antisperm antibodies

Antisperm antibodies can be another problematic condition for some couples. Couples are TTC (trying to conceive) without success. Either they have experienced recurrent miscarriages, or no pregnancy has been achieved. The couple have had all the normal tests performed, to identify any issues in either of them. All test results have come back within normal range. The couple may have been labelled as 'unexplained'. Fertility specialists will not consider further investigations per NICE guidelines, until the couple have had 3 recurrent miscarriages. One of the causes of recurrent miscarriages appears to be when the immune system mistakenly targets sperm in a man's semen as an invader and damages or kills it. Women who have developed antibodies to her partner's sperm may find it useful to have her male partner use condoms for at least 30 days. The sperm antibodies should then decrease, and intercourse without the use of a condom during the time of ovulation may lead to conception. There may be benefits to taking a good vaginal probiotic to raise the levels of good bacteria within this area, such as Optibac.

The case study I mentioned at the beginning was one of these clients. The specialist refused to consider any other factors such as antisperm antibodies attributing to this, even though the client had experienced 3 miscarriages. Once the client admitted to the 3 miscarriages, this was one of my first thoughts along with antiphospholipid syndrome or luteal phase defect. I discussed the idea of any of these conditions being a possibility, and the client agreed to having blood tests performed to identify either of the first 2 conditions whilst we calculated the luteal phase length. There are only a few clinics which will perform the specialist tests for these conditions. The closest to the client was a Dublin clinic who performed the blood tests privately and the result confirmed that she had antiphospholipid syndrome.

Some researchers believe that antiphospholipid syndrome causes tiny blood clots to block the blood supply to the placenta. Others believe that having antiphospholipid syndrome may interfere with the fertilized egg's ability to implant in the lining of the uterus. The client was referred to another consultant in England, who took over her care and monitored her upon conception, with weekly consultations which involved flying to the clinic on the mainland. The client had specific IV solutions administered to help maintain the pregnancy and the blood circulation. Throughout this time, I supported her with fertility reflexology. Working together the client has progressed beyond 15 weeks of pregnancy as I type! There are so many obstacles that couples need to overcome, to achieve a healthy pregnancy! It really is a miracle that it happens!

Non-natural interventions

Throughout, I have talked about the use of more natural approaches for supporting the client, using examples to highlight this. There is of course the need to acknowledge when natural approaches will not achieve the desired outcome, and when invasive or medicated procedures are needed to achieve a pregnancy. These include In Vitro Fertilisation (IVF), Intracytoplasmic Sperm Injection (ICSI), Pre-implantation Genetic Diagnosis (IVF PGD), Frozen Embryo Transfer (FET), IUI (Intra Uterine Insemination), Surgical Sperm Retrieval techniques used to overcome blockages in epididymis or testes, donor eggs/sperm or surrogacy.

As a medical approach, this is a very emotional and hugely physical experience for clients to go through and is an opportunity for therapists to provide support. Clients shouldn't feel that they cannot continue to be supported. On the contrary, I work closely with clients who are undergoing this approach and support them with supplementation and therapies such as fertility reflexology for those going through assisted reproductive techniques (this is taught as part of day 2 of my course, all very organised and step by step techniques for therapists to follow).

Clients will be assessed at the Fertility Clinic and, in conjunction with the couple's medical history and test results, the clinic will determine what approach will be used with the couple. Those clients with a diagnosis of unexplained may be offered IVF, whilst those couples with low sperm count may be offered ICSI. The key difference between IVF and ICSI is how the sperm fertilises the egg.

- In IVF, the egg and sperm (of which there are multiple) are left in a petri dish to fertilise on their own.
- In ICSI, one sperm is directly injected into the egg.

Once the treatment plan has been discussed and arrangements put in place, I ask for a copy of the treatment plan. I also like to know when any amendments are made to the plan. This allows me to adjust the techniques used in line with the client's specific treatment. The plan shows me what medication is being used and when. The dates for commencement of specific medication, the dates of planned scans to assess the ovaries for follicle development or uterine lining thickness, the scheduled days for egg collection and embryo transfer. The information can be interpreted to show me the length of the treatment plan, whether it's a long or short protocol that the clinic are using, whether clients will be placed in a menopausal state for example and the techniques I can use effectively, to support the client at this section of their treatment.

The plan can highlight when the client/s are taking medication to stimulate ovulation and consequently, I know what techniques to use to enhance this part of their treatment, or when I can support them very gently after egg retrieval, or embryo transfer, or during the 'two week wait' when lots of gentle and relaxing support may be required as they anxiously await their pregnancy test day.

I can incorporate visualisation, meditation or EFT for example, ensuring that all therapies are used to enhance the efficacy of the medication of the treatment plan of the clinic. Ideally, it is preferable if these clients attend at least 3 months prior to starting assisted reproductive techniques, as it allows for balancing of hormones, relaxation, dietary review and supplementation, which will strengthen the body in preparation for the next stage of the fertility journey. Regardless of when clients come to me, I support them on their journey to the best of my ability.

About Dorothy Kelly

I've worked in the NHS for 43 years, based now in primary care. I began my career in a women's Hospital in Belfast. It had the first fertility clinic which in the 1970s offered only AID and AIH (artificial insemination by donor or by husband). Following the IVF birth of Louise Brown in 1978, technology advanced dramatically, and the location of the department moved to another major hospital site.

I later had the opportunity to work in the only private fertility clinic in Belfast for a year as the practice manager, where I honed my knowledge and skill in ART, translating it into a reflexology approach which I teach as part of my CPD fertility course. My other Reflexology CPD courses include Maternity and Mental Health support.

I completed naturopathic training through CNM, when they came to Belfast in the late 1990s and subsequently continued to add to my therapy tools with therapies such as Reiki (attuned to Reiki Master - Kokoro Way), Reflexology and numerous CPD courses both in NI/ Ireland and UK. I have since started teaching the Level 5 Reflexology course in Belfast and look to expand into Dublin in the future alongside my husband David who has supported me by teaching the APaP part of the course.

I have to say, working with all the clients I have had the privilege and honour to meet, has brought me joy and happiness, as I share in their journeys and their lives. Wonderful bonds and relationships have developed out of the journeys they have had. Of course there are those with whom I have shared their sorrow and disappointment, but nevertheless these wonderful couples have allowed me into their lives and they have taught me so much and helped me to continue to learn, as I experiment with techniques and continue to read and develop my approach.

To all the students whom I've had the pleasure to meet and remain in contact with, I thank you for putting your trust in me. They have continued to demonstrate, through their case studies and continued fertility reflexology practice, that the methodology works, and they, like me are having great success with their clients. It would be fantastic to document the number of babies this work has helped into the world!

I'm delighted to say an idea which I have been developing for several years has come to fruition. In conjunction with myself, a group of very passionate fertility reflexologists have established an Association of Fertility, which is spreading throughout Northern Ireland and Ireland, with hubs being set up to support both fertility therapists and clients alike. The aim of this is to provide support and knowledge for therapists, as we recognise that the research and medical approaches in the field of fertility keep advancing, and we all need to keep up to date with this, using a variety of media of communication and learning.

As a therapist I have been collecting statistical data to show the importance and relevance of this methodology for supporting clients on their fertility journey. I only began to record numbers from late 2014 even though I've worked with clients from 2010. Since 2014 I have had 275 clients becoming pregnant with a total of 245 live births, which is 88%, an unbelievable and wonderful outcome.

Of the live births 25 births have been from clients having IVF, ICSI or FET. Of the students who replied to my recent request for statistics,

I have also collated 42 sets of results. To date, these students have supported their clients to achieve 286 pregnancies, with 229 live births, 37 of these have been through IVF, ICSI or FET. I am currently waiting on the results of eight pregnancies, with deliveries due in up to six months. Students are similarly waiting on forty-three new births. Fabulous numbers which proves the approach works.

For those interested in attending any of my CPD courses or the Level 5 Reflexology course please visit my website **www.dorothykellyacademyofreflexology.com**. I can be contacted on my facebook page *DorothyKellyFertilityReflexology*, or the Level 5 page *Dorothy Kelly Academy of Reflexology Level 5*.

I travel to England and Ireland at various times of the year to teach CPD as well as holding classes locally in various parts of Northern Ireland. It would be lovely to meet you.

Dorothy Kelly

References

Coenzyme Q10 and male infertility: a meta-analysis
www.ncbi.nlm.nih.gov/pmc/articles/PMC3800531/

Coenzyme Q10 Improves Sperm Parameters, Oxidative Stress Markers and Sperm DNA Fragmentation in Infertile Patients with Idiopathic Oligoasthenozoospermia.
www.ncbi.nlm.nih.gov/pubmed/32009311

Dahl, W. et al. Review of the health benefits of peas (pisum sativum L.). Br J Nutr. 2012;108(1):S3-10

Dehbashi S, Parsanezhad ME, Alborzi S, Zarei A. Effect of clomiphene citrate on endometrium thickness and echogenic patterns. Int J Gynaecol Obstet. 2003;80(1):49–53. doi:10.1016/s0020-7292(02)00341-7

EXAMEN LAB **https://examenlab.com/Defragmentation**

Kar A, Bose A, Das R. Effect of m-xylohydroquinone on the genital organs and fertility of male rats. J. Reprod. Fertility. 1963;(5):77-81.

Lafuente R, González-Comadrán M, Solà I, et al. **www.ncbi. nlm.nih.gov/pmc/articles/PMC3921845/** The role of oxidative stress and antioxidants in male fertility 20/4/2020 or Coenzyme Q10 and male infertility: a meta-analysis. *J Assist Reprod Genet.* 2013;30(9):1147–1156. doi:10.1007/s10815-013-0047-5

www.ncbi.nlm.nih.gov/pmc/articles/PMC5655679/Myo-inositol effects in women with PCOS: a meta-analysis of randomized controlled trials

Lebovitz O, Orvieto R. Treating patients with "thin" endometrium - an ongoing challenge. *Gynecol Endocrinol.* 2014;30(6):409–414. doi :10.3109/09513590.2014.906571

www.pharmanord.co.uk/news/product-information/what-is-omega-7-sba24/Sea Buckthorn

www.sciencedirect.com/topics/neuroscience/phytoestrogens [online] [Accessed19/4/2020]

Starr, J., 2011. *THE EFFECT OF MELATONIN ON THE OVARIES.* [online] Touroscholar.touro.edu. Available at: <https://touroscholar.touro. edu/cgi/viewcontent.cgi?article=1133&context=sjlcas> [Accessed 11 April 2020].

Therapeutic Relationships during Maternity

by Sally Earlam

Therapeutic Relationships during Maternity
by Sally Earlam

Sally Earlam FMAR. BSc. PGCE. (retired RGN)

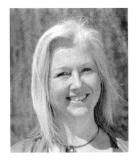

As a reflexologist, working with maternity clients is one of my greatest pleasures and I feel honoured to be part of these special journeys. However there are additional considerations to ensure our pregnant clients' needs are met and a strong therapeutic relationship is built.

For this article I will refer to the foetus as the 'baby'.

Baby brains

A lot of things change when a woman becomes pregnant with some of the most marked changes being the emotional ones. Scientists have now identified that these are largely driven by neurological alterations that occur in the brain that can make a woman obsess and worry about their new little creation. (1)

Under the influence of increasing hormones there are many changes that occur in the brain including in the prefrontal cortex, midbrain and parietal lobes and grey matter becomes more concentrated. These discoveries begin to explain some of the behavioural changes that commonly occur in pregnancy and up to 2 years after the birth of the baby. There is also increased activity in the amygdala, part of the limbic system, which essentially drives our emotional reactions such as fear, anxiety, motivation, affection, empathy etc, and it is this enhanced amygdala that makes new mums hypersensitive to their baby's needs, especially just after the birth.

All of these neurological changes lead to maternal feelings of overwhelming love, fierce protectiveness and worry, and as a result, most pregnant women and new mums want to talk baby and need the space to be able to talk baby. This brings an important consideration for those therapists that want to work in Maternity Reflexology; we need to be in a place where we are able to and want to listen to their baby talk.

It is these emotional and behavioural changes that can affect many, if not all key relationships:

Relationships with their partner

During pregnancy and the first year after the birth, 40-70% of couples report some decline in relationships (2) with the key issues described as:

- Less positive communication – both partners report feeling isolated and less supported
- Tiredness and exhaustion
- Increased conflict e.g. household chores

Of course the same level of neurological changes do not occur in the partner's brains, so you have women who may want to constantly talk baby and feel the partner is not interested in the baby (they are, but not to the same level) and the partner who feels their relationship is being neglected.

If these types of concerns are raised by your client, then reassure her it is normal. Encourage her to talk to, and listen to her partner and maybe suggest she shares her hopes and dreams and encourages her partner to share theirs as this may help initiate some two-way positive communication. But perhaps best of all, suggest she tries to arrange some quality time for them together, doing something they both enjoy, as a reminder of why they fell in love in the first place.

Relationships with friends and family

This can be a trying time for many of those longstanding relationships that have previously been a key part of your client's support network, there are two possible scenarios that can take place with family or friends:

■ **They start to withdraw from the relationship** as they may feel excluded or jealous as they are at a different stage in their lives and don't want to listen to 'baby talk'. It could even be that they have had issues with conception and it is too painful for them.

Reassure your client that friendships can sometimes adapt or come back later in life and new friendships will be made. You could suggest she looks for antenatal classes in her local area to meet with other mums-to-be.

■ **They offer unwanted advice or criticism**. Pregnancy seems to bring with it plenty of 'advice' from others whether asked for or not.

Reassure her that it is OK to say that some decisions need to be made by her and her partner and they will decide what is right for them.

Relationships with their baby

This is a time when your client is developing a completely new relationship and the changes that occur in the brain are similar to the changes that occur when you fall in love – only this time thoughts are dominated by the baby not the partner. Of course in all of this the mother has one very willing audience who will never tire of the baby talk – and that is the baby. Babies are thought to recognise the mother's voice from around 26 weeks and the sound of her voice will calm the baby. Unborn babies clearly respond to different vibrations and sounds with changes in their heart rate and movement patterns, and are particularly responsive to the sound of their mother's voice (3).

Encourage the mother to talk to their baby. Talking and singing to their bump can be a lovely way to start building a relationship with their unborn baby and can benefit them as well as their baby.

Relationships with themselves

All of the swirling hormones and changes in the brain lead to many unfamiliar feelings for the woman – they can be on an emotional rollercoaster and find it hard to comprehend how they can be laughing one minute and crying the next. How they see themselves as a worker, a friend, a partner, a mother to be is changing and can also bring up memories of how they were parented – and these can be good or bad.

Remember, this is a time when anxiety is more common, you can reassure them this is normal to have worries but if you have concerns that their anxiety is affecting their everyday life encourage them to talk to their midwife or GP. It is also possible to refer yourself without seeing a GP if you live in England through the NHS website. (4)

Building a relationship of trust with your client

The Therapeutic Relationship is something we are all familiar with but it is worth reminding ourselves as we can slip into bad habits, especially when we have been seeing a client for a while. The key elements of the therapeutic relationship are:

- an ongoing relationship between a therapist and the client that is established to support the client's therapeutic goals;
- it is a relationship of support and is a helpful resource for the client;
- a healthy therapeutic relationship includes, trust, respect, safety, authenticity, acceptance, empathy, and collaborative agreement.

So the client remains in the centre of everything we do, if you are trying to make the decision of whether to share your experiences ask yourself: am I going to tell the story because I think it will benefit the client? In which case share. Or is it just because you want to talk about it? In which case do not share.

A good therapeutic relationship is essential for retaining clients, it improves outcomes, adds to their motivation and promotes their disclosure. It is not just about what we do as a reflexologist but who we are with our clients. We need to ensure our clients have the experience of a warm encounter and they need to feel relaxed, listened to, able to speak freely and perhaps most importantly in maternity they need to feel safe – as this is a time when women can feel vulnerable.

Our aim is always to build a relationship of trust – so how can this be achieved?

First impressions

You have only 7 seconds to make a first impression. Within these 7 seconds of meeting, people will have a solid impression of who you are and some research suggests a tenth of a second is all it takes to start determining traits such as trustworthiness (5). Once they have made their judgement it is then very difficult to change their minds.

So how do we make the most of the 7 seconds?

- Dress appropriately – smart and clean – you will be judged on how you look before you even speak.
- Greet each client with a genuine warm smile as it sends the message that you are trustworthy and approachable.
- Shake hands as touch tells them you care.
- Maintain good eye contact.
- Speak slowly and clearly as it sends the message you are articulate and intelligent.
- Keep good posture, with your shoulders back and your head held high, as this makes you appear and feel more confident.

Making the most of your verbal communication

Once your client has settled onto a chair or couch then this is when what you say becomes more important. On first meeting, make sure you share your experience and skill set and show your passion for reflexology. Being passionate about a subject is one of the biggest factors for inspiring, energising and influencing others.

Other tips:

- **Tell a story** – as these reach into hearts and minds and will be better remembered e.g. "I had a client who......".
- **Keep the client at the centre** – everything is client focused.
- **Don't get stuck in therapy mode** – this means empathy not sympathy – nodding sympathetically or reaffirming that something is terrible just keeps them stuck in their mud – acknowledge that you understand and try to reframe their challenges into potential opportunities.
- **Give them hope** – even a smidgen, as long as it is realistic, can help them see that there may just be a way that they can feel better. Giving clients hope improves outcomes.
- **Give information** – don't criticise or tell them what to do as nobody likes this!

- **Show genuine appreciation, admiration and acknowledge their growth** – as this helps build self-esteem.

Building the therapeutic relationship in pregnancy

Probably the most important consideration here is that pregnant women need to know that they are in safe and knowledgeable hands; Mums-to-be can feel vulnerable and need additional reassurance. So be explicit and tell them about your experience, and share your knowledge – if you don't know something, say you don't know but you will find out. It is also worth learning about the changes that occur in pregnancy and about baby development if you are not familiar with these.

Be vocal about the importance of comfort and safety e.g. "It is really important that you feel comfortable during your treatment, so if at any point you feel you would like to change position please let me know" or "I am just going to sit you up slowly and we will make sure you feel OK before you stand up".

Other considerations

- Be genuinely interested in their pregnancy.
- Give them time to talk about their pregnancy and worries.
- Ask questions to show you care – ask about their partner, work, parents etc.
- Have professional, good quality support materials e.g. AoR Maternity leaflets.

And to finish – be creative!

There is no magic formula for developing the perfect Therapeutic Relationship so try to be creative. Don't get stuck in a rut and try mixing things up as repetitive experiences can lose their capacity to help change and growth. This may mean changing the way you ask questions, changing your reflexology sequence or even moving your treatment room around. Think about your practice and how you make your clients feel special.

About Sally Earlam. – Maternity Specialist and Head of Training and Education for the Association of Reflexologists. Sally also runs CPD courses in small groups in a warm, friendly and supportive environment in SE London – www.sallyearlam.co.uk.

1. Swain JE, Lorberbaum JP, Kose S, Strathearn L.. Brain basis of early parent-infant interactions: psychology, physiology, and in vivo functional neuroimaging studies.. J Child Psychol Psychiatry. 2007 Mar-Apr;48(3-4):262-87.

2. Shapiro, A.F. and Gottman, J.M., 2005. Effects on Marriage of a Psycho- Communicative-Educational Intervention With Couples Undergoing the Transition to Parenthood, Evaluation at 1-Year Post Intervention. Journal of Family Communication 5, 1–24.

3. Voegtline KM et al. Near-term fetal response to maternal spoken voice. Infant Behav Dev 2013;36:526-33.

4. https://beta.nhs.uk/find-a-psychological-therapies-service/

5. https://www.forbes.com/sites/serenitygibbons/2018/06/19/you-have-7-seconds-to-make-a-first-impression-heres-how-to-succeed/#4034d1b56c20

Reflexology as a Communication Tool Between the Mother and her Unborn Baby

by Heinrike Bergmans

Reflexology as a Communication Tool Between the Mother and her Unborn Baby
by Heinrike Bergmans

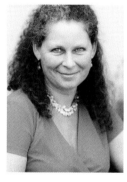

As I am writing this chapter, we are in the midst of covid-19. My heart goes out to all the pregnant women and their partners. Pregnancy itself is already an intense process of transformation for the baby, the mother and the father. With the lockdown, many 'normal' contacts are now only done at a physical distance, often online and this causes more stressful situations. Feeling safe in your own body is key to developing a good sense of safety with the unborn baby, and in that regard, as a learning process for the baby to feel safe inside itself.

1 Prenatal imprints influence life

From the moment the egg-cell of a mother merges with the sperm-cell of a father, a chain reaction happens. Rapid multiplications of the first cell, called a zygote, start building your body. These multi potential cells have a tipping point at which they start to specialise and fulfil a very specific role. Some cells will start building and preparing the implantation into the endometrium, others will start building the 3-germ layers out of which organs and body parts will grow.

In embryology we find the blueprint of how our bodies are built. Every single one of us has built their body themselves. The role of the mother is providing a healthy, safe, and sustainable environment in which this process gets all the necessary nutrients and support on a physical, emotional, mental and spiritual level. Our human biology is built in such an ingenious way that the view of a pregnant woman on the world will prepare the unborn life to live in it. And this is the case in both thriving and in surviving conditions.

2 Beyond the physical body

As human beings we are so much more than our body. Our sensory system gives us an impression of how the world looks. And as our eyes can not see ultraviolet light and our ears can only hear within a certain range, there is an entire world we are not able to see, hear, smell, feel and taste. Yet all these other frequencies do exist.

In the book 'Vibrational Medicine', Dr. Richard Gerber describes a multi-layer human anatomy based upon different frequencies and explained by the Tiller model. All these different layers of our being, also called subtle bodies, co-exist at the same time and in the same place. In figure 1 below, you see the frequency model of subtle bodies in a human being by W. Tiller, Ph.D.

We express our soul on earth through a physical body. Beyond that body there is an ethereal body. The meridian system is connecting the physical body with our ethereal body. So meridians have a physical and ethereal dimension. The ethereal body has chakras that connect to the meridian system, the nervous system and the hormonal glands. The plane in which the chakras exist is the ethereal. And from the ethereal plane they have an influence on the physical plane. The next frequency spectrum is the astral body that has a very subtle energy in a higher energetic frequency than the ethereal. Here our emotions reside and are the mechanisms for intangible awareness. It offers the possibility to go beyond time and space and have a look at

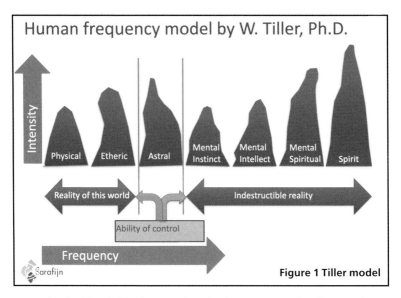

Figure 1 Tiller model

your physical body like in people who have a near-death experience and sense themselves floating above their body.

Beyond the astral body is the mental body where the mental beliefs reside on an instinctive, intellectual and spiritual level and finally the causal body. Probably there are even more frequencies that we are yet to discover. Although we can distinguish these different bodies, they cannot be separated as they co-exist at the same time and in the same space.

The model shows that the frequencies of the physical and ethereal body create our reality in this world. The ethereal body provides the physical body with the necessary energy to exist in the physical world. When the physical body dies, the ethereal body dies as well and returns through the process of dissolving back into the free energy of the universe. As the frequencies become higher, there lies a reality that goes beyond time and space, creating a framework where past, present and future are present at the same time, as well as space, being an omni space.

If one is not aware of a world outside of time and space as we are often taught by our earthly parents and society, there is also no awareness of the astral body and beyond. Everything that has to do with a soul and a Self with a capital S then sounds weird, bizarre, unearthly and out of our control. By becoming aware of these frequencies, the world and its meaning suddenly becomes wider. It is the discovery of new dimensions, possibilities and ways of being.

3 Conscious pregnancy

A pregnancy is an incredibly special process. The presence of the incoming form of consciousness literally pushes the mother from within into her physical, ethereal, astral, mental and causal body. Since this is so for 38 weeks, 24 hours a day, this is a very intense process, which can be experienced consciously or unconsciously. Not only does this affect the system of the future mother, but also that of the future father and grandparents, the circle of friends and working environment. In short, everything in the immediate surroundings. The more conscious a mother, and the people surrounding her, can experience a pregnancy, the more the world in which the baby will be born is open to embracing and raising the new life in a very conscious way.

In different cultures we find data about contact with unborn children long before they were conceived. Currently, this is becoming more and more tangible, visible and especially discussable in the Western world. In the book by Anne Hubbel Maiden and Edie Farwell "The Tibetan Art of Parenting" it is described how women within Tibetan Buddhism often receive the announcement of their unborn child in their dreams. This is also found in Christian faith. Mary received the conception of her son Jesus announced by the Angel Gabriel. More and more women in the West experience this in their dreams as well as in their daily consciousness. Rosemarijn Roes, a Dutch author writes about this in her book "Mama, are you listening?". She explains how the unborn children guide their mothers to her so she can pass on the message the children have to give to their mothers who are not yet able to listen to their unborn children themselves or are afraid to accept that they can.

Before conception, children can be sensed in the ethereal aura of the mother by the mother. With my third son Neo (2006) I had telepathic contact two years before he was born, which was also very strong during pregnancy. On a regular basis we communicated what was going. Several of my clients can feel their unborn children in their aura before conception. The broader the consciousness, the more consciously you can experience everything in your daily life. I strongly believe that children who are seen, felt and communicated with before conception and during pregnancy, start to develop a good connection with their astral, mental and causal body. And as pregnancy doesn't just happens to you, a mother is learning to connect to these levels due to the resonance of her unborn baby. This wonderful picture of Alex Grey shows a glimpse of the different layers in the subtle world.

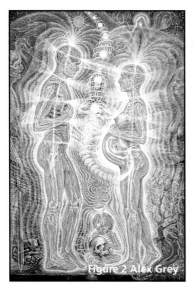

Figure 2 Alex Grey

Sometimes, growing in consciousness requires a slow pass to take it all in. We learn to become a multi-dimensional being through our children, both our born and unborn children. Not every soul you feel needs to be born, sometimes feeling its presence is enough to continue the soul's and your own growth.

How can you picture this? Unborn souls or children are energetically as real as people, but without a physical and ethereal body (that is why they also incarnate, namely they become flesh and blood). Once you get familiar with this kind of energy, you can talk with them just like you do with people but in a telepathic way. They carry their own information field with them based on their mental and causal body. Depending on your own sensitivity, you will be able to see them, hear them, feel them, or just know they are there.

On a soul level, parents and children match on a quest to bringing more consciousness into this world. By opening themselves to the unborn baby, by longing for it, by letting it be born, parents can reconnect to their own higher energies and will gradually or suddenly make a voyage of creating a new personality.

The wonderful thing is that for every parent there is a combination with an unborn soul. It is tailor-made for all parties. From the moment the first desire begins to grow in parents, an unborn soul will respond to this and begin to compact itself energetically, i.e. be more and more present in the aura of the parents. This can be felt by both the father and the mother. Even before there is physical conception, the energetic body of the mother may be pregnant and feel physically pregnant (swollen breasts and belly).

4 Reflexology as a communication tool to connect and feel safe

When I started learning reflexology, I was trained to follow a certain sequence on the feet, foot by foot and a mindset of physical ailments. Gradually this changed into tailored treatments adapted to the specific needs of the person in front of me and at the same time, monitoring their mental and emotional state. Besides using grips and holds with lots of movements, I started to experiment with grips that are more static and energetic. Being extremely sensitive, I learned that very often before my clients could sense anything, I already did, which was very confusing in the beginning. It took me a while to understand how I could fine-tune so that the sensing of my clients (maybe you call them patients but in Belgium we are not allowed to do so) became a learning tool in reconnecting with their own body. So if you feel a bit dazzled in the beginning when you start working this way, feel happy. It is an indication that you are on the right path.

From there I evolved into coaching through the feet. A few clients triggered me as their mindset would immediately undo the work that was done on their feet. So, if I was able to integrate their mental mindset in my work, then an extra impulse could be used for transformation.

Today, as a coach and reflexologist I see myself as a facilitator monitoring the process that is on the one hand happening inside, the reaction on a physical, emotional, mental and spiritual level and on the other hand, the process with me as the facilitator. The word participant is justified because at any moment, only they can truly intervene, monitored by the facilitator, but only they can regain control when they lose it, only they can release emotions and change their beliefs when they are ready to do so. In that regard, reflexology is a communication tool to support the process, especially in offering safety and building body awareness.

With SARAFIJN I developed a reflexology based coaching technique that offers participants the potential to tune in with their astral, mental and causal body. Tuning in to these higher frequencies enables emotional release from beyond time and space and the possibility to change your own mental belief system. As you are reading this chapter, I am working together with a psychologist who is taking qEEGs before and after sessions to see what is actually happening in the brain. As we get more sessions registered, it starts to show that the Sarafijn Basic Technique (SBT) has a deep impact on the delta brain waves. The results of these registrations will be presented at the upcoming RiEN conference in Paris 2021.

SARAFIJN is the acronym for:

- **S**afety - feeling safe makes one open up to the world
- **A**wareness - being aware of how a process works
- (Emotional) **R**esilience - learning how to switch between emotions
- (Mental) **A**gility - learning how to work with potential paths in life
- **F**ocus - training the ability to align intention, attention and action
- **I**nner State - training the ability to amplify using emotions
- **J**oin - connecting with like-minded people
- **N**ever-ending - as one step is taken, another will follow in a never-ending process

The trinity grip is the basic grip that is used within Sarafijn Basic Technique and Sarafijn Coaching. It offers the possibility to go beyond time and space when properly performed. Essential is the body awareness of the facilitator whether you are a reflexologist or body therapist. Your awareness will function as a tuning fork, resonating safety and holding space. And as you get more familiar and more powerful in this, your participants, supported by the trinity hold, will do so too. If you would like to have a look at the effect, go to the YouTube video via this link:**https://youtu.be/lDvUrLeKqDI**.

4.1 The Trinity Grip

The basis for this grip is the Shuni mudra whereby the thumb touches the middle finger without adding any pressure. Have a look at figure 3. This mudra stands for patience and the power of discernment, and for building up the courage to help you fulfil your own responsibilities. A mudra is a hand gesture used in Buddhist sculptures and paintings. Mudras have an influence on the flow of energy and on a person's mood. The trinity grip is a grip that connects to the different layers of our multi-dimensional energy system all the way into the physical level. They are the reactions within the physical level that are used to monitor and create balance and connection.

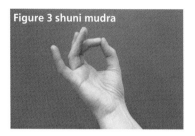

Figure 3 shuni mudra

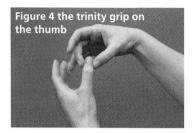

Figure 4 the trinity grip on the thumb

Have a look at figure 4 of the trinity grip on the thumb of your own hand. That way you can start to experiment right away on yourself. The starting position of the trinity grip is formed by placing your thumb of your working hand on the thumb of the hand being worked and your middle finger on the opposite side of the thumb of the hand being worked. Now invite the energy to flow through both fingers.

This grip is used to achieve harmony in the following three parts of a constellation.

- Part 1: Focus on the thumb or the middle finger of the working hand until a change can be observed. This can be a throbbing feeling, or a sensation of warmth, movement or tingling.
- Part 2: Now focus on the other finger and feel whether there is a change, then observe the rhythm and the intensity.
- Part 3: Finally, focus simultaneously on the thumb and the finger as they form a unity. Continue with the same grip until the rhythm of the pulsation in the middle finger and the thumb is the same.

A deeper way to sense the power of this grip, is by looking in your hand for a sour or painful spot. Once you have found it, rest the thumb of your working hand on this spot and put your middle finger on the opposite side. Make sure you only touch - the nails should not turn white due to too much pressure. Follow again the three parts as discussed above. Once you feel balance, push deeper into the tissue and sense for the tension you observed earlier. How does it feel now?

4.2 The Bi-manual Trinity Grip

The bi-manual trinity grip is used when working on others and performed with both hands simultaneously. When applied, it works as a triple system done three times.

Left foot (system 1)

- **Part 1:** Focus on the thumb or the middle finger of the working hand until a change can be observed. This can be a throbbing feeling, or a sensation of warmth, movement or tingling.
- **Part 2:** Now focus on the other finger and feel whether there is a change, then observe the rhythm and the intensity.
- **Part 3:** Finally, focus simultaneously on the thumb and the finger as they form a unity. Continue with the same grip until the rhythm of the pulsation in the middle finger and the thumb is the same. The inside and outside of the left foot are now balanced.

Right foot (system 2)

- **Part 1:** Focus on the thumb or the middle finger of the working hand until a change can be observed. This can be a throbbing feeling, or a sensation of warmth, movement or tingling.
- **Part 2:** Now focus on the other finger and feel whether there is a change, then observe the rhythm and the intensity.
- **Part 3:** Finally, focus simultaneously on the thumb and the finger as they form a unity. Continue with the same grip until the rhythm of the pulsation in the middle finger and the thumb is the same. The inside and outside of the right foot are now balanced.

Both foot (system 3)

- **Part 1:** Focus on the left foot and the pulsation between the thumb and the middle finger of the working hand. Hold until the pulsation of both is the same.

- **Part 2:** Now focus on the right foot and the pulsation between the thumb and the middle finger of the working hand. Hold until the pulsation of both is the same.
- **Part 3:** Finally, hold the grip until the rythmn of the pulsation of the trinity grip on the left foot is the same as in the right foot. The left side and the right side of the body are now balanced.

When you use the bi-manual trinity grip on the pelvis reflex, you are not only supporting the pelvis, but at the same time also chakra 1 and the entire spine. In haptonomy*, supporting a newborn baby by supporting the pelvis, is giving the baby, (although it is not able to sit upright yet) the support to do so. The gesture and the presence in this gesture enables the baby to sense what it is to feel and sit upright. With the same intention, this bi-manual trinity grip should be performed.

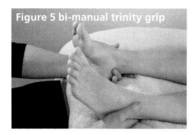

Figure 5 bi-manual trinity grip

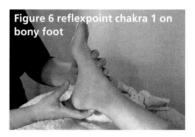

Figure 6 reflexpoint chakra 1 on bony foot

*Haptonomy is a method to develop a loving relationship with your baby throughout pregnancy. It is based on the relation of tenderness that exists between the baby, mother and father/partner. Its principal objective is to develop a sense of security and autonomy in each of these three partners by taking into consideration their specific psycho-effective needs.

5 Examples of working with pregnant women and unborn children

Working with pregnant women is a privilege. Pregnancy is an incredibly special moment in a lifetime where a new life is building itself cell by cell and at the same time, a woman is transforming into a mother.

5.1 Past high emotional memory triggered in the present

During a maternity reflexology training, a midwife who was having visiting hours next door asked for help. A first-time mother who came during visiting hours was convinced that her child was going to die and expressed high levels of fear and anxiety. The midwife had already put her on the monitor, and everything appeared to be fine with the baby. Because the midwife was convinced that we could support her with reflexology, she was brought into our group.

Step 1: Safety and holding space

As the woman lay down on the massage bed, she consented that all the students could stay present and observe what was happening.

To offer safety, the bi-manual trinity hold (figure 5) was performed on her heels reflecting the pelvis area. This hold simulates the supporting of the pelvis and the entire spine so the person laying down can feel as if they are upright.

At the same time, she was invited to bring her attention inside her heels. After several attempts she said that she could not get out of her head. She was convinced that her baby was going to die and kept being worried about it.

High emotional reactions prevent us from using the frontal cortex and use our mental abilities to switch focus. So not being able to use this, the best approach is using the body to bring the mind into the presence.

I asked her to make contact with her belly by putting her hands on her belly. And to feel the warmth of her hands on her belly, making small movements so she could feel this.

When people are coming out of an emotional reaction or out of their head, as a reflexologist you can sense the change in general tention in the feet. Besides that, facial expressions change and become softer as well as the intonation of the voice.

As she proceeded, she was invited to feel for her baby in her belly. And so she did. She could feel the baby moving in the abdomen. The baby was cooperating from the inside as lower muscular tensions provide more space for movement. Then I asked her what she was afraid of. She repeated that she was afraid that her baby would die but she had no idea where this feeling was coming from.

Step 2: Differentiating

Again, I asked her to make contact with the baby and feel what it was like. She could feel that her baby was okay, but that something else on her belly gave a sensation of tension.

Now being in a safe mode, she was able to observe in a more neutral way. That way she could become aware that there was a field of tension that was not related to the baby but that was tangible in her own body.

I asked her if it would be OK for her to investigate this feeling a bit more. And as she consented, I asked her to invite the entire information field that was attached to it, to come out and show itself. Meanwhile she was still supported by the bi-manual trinity hold on her heels.

By inviting the information field to show itself, the person is able to look at the situation from an observer position. That way, although emotions can be felt, there is an overview of the situation and more factors can be taken into consideration.

Step 3: Emotional release/mental agility

Eventually, the situation that revealed itself to her was the death of her mother. She missed her so much and tears started to come. She was incredibly sorry that she couldn't share her pregnancy and childbirth with her. Another level of grief was touched and released.

As she saw her mother, she was invited to say to her what she still wanted to say. So she did, and by doing so she gave herself the possibility to rewrite her own memory. Loss changed into sharing, releasing grief, and opening to joy for the unborn life.

The suppressed grief of the death of her mother was mirrored into the possible death of her baby. In Sarafijn Basic Technique and Coaching we call this mirror communication. By allowing the grief and the loss, she was able to release the tension in her belly area.

In this process the bi-manual trinity hold was changed into a bi-manual connection between the reflex of tension on the belly and the reflex of chakra 1.

Step 4: Reconnection to the body

Finally, she was invited to say goodbye to her mother and bring her attention back to her belly. She could feel that the tension was gone and that there was more space. She could also feel that the baby was moving and that it was alright to be joyful about the coming birth. She also understood that giving in to joy would express respect for life itself and that her mother would have wanted this as well for her.

Strong positive emotions such as joy can evoke also suppressed emotions and at the same time, suppressed emotions complicate the free sensing of positive emotions.

5.2 Working with children in the aura

Agnes felt incredibly anxious about the idea of having another child. She did not know where this feeling was coming from, but it was there, and she did not feel comfortable with it. As this was limiting her daily functioning, she asked to explore this feeling.

Step 1: Safety and holding space

We started with the bi-manual trinity grip on the pelvis reflex. As she started to feel the energy flow inside her body, she became calmer and more focused. She was more connected with her own body and spirit. As she closed her eyes, she could see and sense an unborn child in her aura and made connection with it.

When the participant starts to feel the energy flow, they are entering a stage of going beyond time and space. The bi-manual trinity hold supports them in doing so. It enables it and at the same time it offers safety, knowing that one is not alone in this journey of new explorations.

Step 2: Differentiating

By connecting to the unborn child in her aura, she opened to new parts of information about herself. As she started to communicate with this child, she was able to discover that her fear had another origin. It was not about having another child; it was about living her true potential in this world. This child was a child part of her that wanted to express itself.

Within the perception of every day, projections of own thoughts and feelings are made upon others and other things. Going beyond time and space puts a different perspective on things.

Step 3: Emotional release/mental agility

This insight touched her very deeply. She allowed herself to release emotions of fear and failure. At that moment in time, she was on sick leave. She had a strong desire to change jobs but did not know what the future would bring. Her confusion about how to raise a child on her own, changed into wondering what kind of new job she would like to do.

When emotions start to release, a new potential emerges that has been blocked up to that time. Also, this can be overwhelming. The important thing at this stage is to allow and give safety to exploring the new and staying aware that this still can trigger old emotions. If so, allow these emotions to be as sliding doors. In the end, they will fully release.

Step 4: Reconnection to the body

As she was able to release the emotions, things became very clear for her. She felt how right it was for her to make a career and go for the next steps. With this new feeling and view upon her life, we again connected to the body, sensing if the flow of energy was flowing everywhere or if there were still new areas of potential to be discovered. As everything was flowing now, we ended the session.

I would rather not speak about blockages in words as that is what they do, they block. I speak and think in terms of potential. Where is a potential frozen and ready for release? In a session, more than one potential can pop up but not always.

6 Evolution

Over the course of years and the combination of reflexology, coaching and training body awareness, I enjoy the evolution I see. More and more women start to understand that pregnancy is far more than getting a baby. I have the privilege to work with women and men who want to prepare themselves before conception, releasing old emotions and thoughts, working very consciously on their own awareness.

I believe that children that are received this way are souls who are willing and ready to take the next step we need on earth to uplight awareness. I am grateful to be part of this process, knowing at the same time that I'm still learning a lot and hope to continue to do so. If you sense that you resonate with this idea too, do follow that feeling. The world needs it. I wish you the best of luck!

About Heinrike Bergmans

In September 2002 I started my reflexology training and attended my first RiEN Conference in Italy in May 2003. A new world opened up and it felt like home. Eager to learn more, I trained with Susanne Enzer, Griet Rondel, Peter Lund Frandsen and, Dorthe Krogsgaard, Martine Faure-Alderson, Shmuel Zaïdel, Dwight Byers and Hanne Marquardt and many others.

To give reflexology a legal place in Belgian society, I co-founded the Belgian professional reflexology organisation BeVo and was chair for 7 years, co-founded 'Integratieve Reflexologie', a reflexology school and co-worked with teachers across Europe.

Currently in my daily work I combine reflexology with transformational and body awareness coaching, training self regulation and co-regulation along with career coaching. I believe that in tomorrow's world, a next generation can be trained in self-regulation by the mother for before conception and during pregnancy, supported by the father, the family and new systems. Children that are seen, felt and have dialogues in this way, have a better body connection. And at the same time, all of us have imprints from the past. Transforming them offers the world in which we live a future based upon thriving instead of surviving.

My three pregnancies, a near death experience and my background in business engineering pushed me to look for energy flow optimisations by understanding how different systems co-exist and work together on both a tangible and intangible level. Covid-19 offered me the opportunity to start teaching online and training hands-on off-line. If this resonates with you to learn, to organise, to exchange or to pioneer, feel free to contact or connect with me.

Heinrike can be contacted at:

www.sarafijn.be
heinrike@sarafijn.be
www.facebook.com/sarafijn
www.linkedin.com/in/heinrike-bergmans-b1821aa/

A Quantum welcome for the Incoming Soul

by Jenni Tribe

A Quantum welcome for the Incoming Soul
by Jenni Tribe

Introduction

There has never been a more important time to realise that change is necessary in order to address the current climate of fear and loss of control on a global scale for the survival of the human race.

With increasing restrictions on our freedoms of speech, movement, and autonomy, the world is changing daily if not hourly. This is nothing new as we remember the uprising of civilisations of eons past. However, the global challenges are generating enormous shifts in the Earth's frequency which affects our own vitality and challenges our congruence.

This chapter is not intended to be political or judgemental but an urgent plea to wake up and realise the magnitude of this opportunity for cataclysmic expansion and development on a personal and universal dimension.

In this chapter I will be discussing how our existence depends on the vibrational connection to our environment and how vital our bonding with our mother affects our physiological and neurological development; how the lack and deprivation of love and nurturing affects our self-perceptions and self-worth and our perceived place in society, resulting in adverse outcomes and further parenting issues. We need to disrupt the cycle.

I will discuss why we need to get it right when it comes to conscious parenting in an ideal world, supporting loving conceptions of wanted children and how to resolve traumatic upbringings. To become the best practitioners, we must recognise the need for our own personal reflection and development order to enhance our own experiential learning while empowering those we support. I share with you some aspects of maternity reflexology to incorporate in your sessions and greater insight into an expanded awareness for implementing more vibrational energy work into the current techniques you may be using.

In an ideal world

In an idyllic world all babies are born equal and from an act of unconditional love, not as an act of fixing or forcing a relationship, not from an act of violence or self-sustaining abuse out of a disconnection to source identity, for example. In this ultimate world of choice, enlightenment and empowerment the parents, particularly the mother (for this chapter I will be referring to the vessel of creation and carrier of the pregnancy of the incoming souls as 'mother'), will have chosen her time to conceive and the partner she wishes to unite with and in a frequency of unconditional love, to consciously couple and conceive. The manifestation of the incoming soul energy amalgamating into physical matter may occur in the first few moments after conjoining of the spermatic DNA to the ovum. As we will discover later it seems the outdated masculine-biased view that the strongest swimmer gets there first may be mythical as it appears the ovum influences the selection of her own suitor.

A friend recalls that at the time of climax he felt his future son connect with him and drawn into existence. He knew his wife was pregnant before she did. He continues to cherish a very close bond with his son.

The Himba tribe in Namibia, South Africa, considers the day the mother conceives the thought of having a child as the day of celebration rather than the birthday. She will take herself off into the wilderness and download the song of the incoming souls which she then teaches to her husband who will learn the song for the mating and this song will be sung at all significant developmental stages of their life. This may seem rather romantic. Alas the life of a Himba tribeswoman is strenuous and arduous and all the female and male members of the tribe are circumcised, among other strict traditions. (1)

Everything is energy. We are but a physical representation of all that surrounds us and passes and interacts with us and remains in a constant state of flow. Research shows that our thoughts create change in the morphic fields around us as the thought causes molecules to interact and exchange and affect the frequencies in our environment. Remember the jars of cooked rice experiment, one labelled 'hate' and verbally abused frequently while the other was labelled 'love' and adored? Unsurprisingly, that which was bullied, rotted far more quickly than that which was nurtured with vibes of affection and kindness. So how will an incoming soul react to a conception of remorseless regret and an upbringing of hate and trauma? Sue Gerhardt's work shows that the prefrontal cortex in the brain is stimulated and develops an empathy to others when love is given to new babies and the neglect of such increases the responses of anxiety, insensitivity and aggression and a reduced immune response. (2) Have you seen the video of a two year old that recognises a poorly puppy that needs rescuing and demonstrates an innate wisdom that the dog calmly responds to? Parents who realise the importance of relationships will raise connected children.

So how do we know how to react? We learn behaviours from those we live with and are exposed to. Our amygdalae control the hypothalamus, pituitary, adrenal (HPA) axis and overstimulation of our fear responses causes us to desensitise and dumb down our reactions, losing empathy for others. The recent introduction of holding thermometer 'guns' to a masked child's head before admission to school certainly raised my heckles, did it yours? What will this desensitisation lead to?

Dr Thomas R Verny, pre and perinatal psychiatrist and leading expert, explains that babies react to external stimuli, shouting, loud noises, from 6 months gestation onwards and you can find an ultrasound video demonstrating this. I found it quite alarming to watch this beautiful soul jump at the shock of the sound of smashing glass and external shouting, responding to the sudden increase in mum's stress hormones.

Where do we make the conclusions whether something is safe or not? We learn it and our beliefs from those we trust, rightly or wrongly. The brainwaves of our development cause us to be programmable from the beginning of life, exposed to the variety of energetic vibrational rhythms surrounding us at all times. As a new-born, our brainwaves are delta waves and every reaction, thought and perception will influence the construction of the very cells of the newly developing infant's brain. The peaks of the brain folds (gyri) and the troughs (sulci) start developing from 10 weeks gestation and most will take shape in the third trimester between 28-38 weeks and then continue lifelong as the brain develops further connections. The neural pathways can adapt to what we think about most and this plasticity creates a golden opportunity for change: what we used to think about most that didn't serve us in good light, can be adapted and resolved. Yes, trauma can be loved out of us! I use the term 'good light' with intention as this is crucial to our understanding of just what energy we are running on - solar energy. In reality, we are all energised stardust reacting in response to our environment, powered by the Sun.

By the age of 2 the infant becomes aware of themselves as separate from mum and regards themselves as 'me', having previously perceived themselves as part of mother even after birth (theta brainwaves). The beliefs of the family set up, role models and relationship qualities, rightly and wrongly, are learned before 6-7 years of age (alpha) and then life is taken and lived according to these personal laws (beta).

Dr Bruce Lipton's work with his 'Biology of Belief' is a ground-breaking realisation that our reality depends entirely on whether we feel we are surviving or thriving in our personal reality. When we feel we are safe, our physiology acts accordingly, we repair and recuperate while asleep and awake refreshed and our parasympathetic and autonomic nervous systems keep us ticking over and our cells replenish and rejuvenate constantly. However, if we consistently feel unsafe and threatened by the stressful demands of our everyday life, the mechanisms that are designed for a short, swift reaction to save us from risk become excessively familiar and our ability to restore the status quo becomes impaired. We are all familiar with the signs of fright and flight- the same as a triple espresso: heart rate escalates and respiratory rate increases in a bid to detoxify, pupils dilate to see more clearly, the gut purges and we feel energised and jittery, muscles primed for a rapid exit. This peak response passes and once the toxic caffeine metabolises and our systems recover, our gastrointestinal system can start digesting and absorbing again. This is why when we are treating our clients, a familiar indication of a state of relaxation is that the belly rumbles and the bowels develop a new 'language of release'. If you are in somatic resonance, then you may experience sympathetic belching and yawning. Exercise is helpful in the treatment of anxiety and depression as the movement assists the self-regulation of excess cortisol and epinephrine levels hence the term "walking it off".

A brilliant book by Robert Sapolsky: " Why zebras don't get ulcers" explains the damaging effects of relentless stress and our hardening resistance to undoing the harm caused by chronic hyper inflammatory states if we don't practice relaxation and allow ourselves to unwind. Research also shows that if we harden our hearts emotionally then we actualise physical hardening of our coronary tissues in a condition called heart lock where the coronary arteries actually stenose. Fortunately, we have also discovered that a change in mindset can reverse this dis-ease. And there we have it: the whole premise that illness is actually dis-ease, an imbalance of homeostasis, a disorder of being well.

When things go wrong and we lose connection

As the germ layers of the blastocyst and the placenta establish themselves in the order of development of the newly conceived entity, any trauma and disruption of the delicate balance of harmony is stored and recorded in the resonance of these developing and multiplying cells. These are like scratches on the surface of a DVD disc. The playback is going well but every now and then there appears interference, a skip, a blip. It may pass, though if overwhelming, the whole thing gets stuck and the whole thing is ejected. As it is, for our development. Ever wondered at a tadpole or growing leaf - how the cells know what shape to grow into? How it forms and changes? It's called a genetic blueprint, a predestined pattern of energy. We are a holonomic blueprint and with the right energy and environment we evolve and adapt with full potential but with a destructive force and persistent abuse, our demeanour becomes challenged and we won't grow properly emotionally, physically or spiritually. The earlier they occur and the deeper the scratches become, the harder we struggle to play on without feeling triggered. Then we practice avoidance in order to protect ourselves from further unpleasant exposure and experiences. Maternal stress has been linked with an increase in Schizophrenia in boys of mothers experiencing PTSD and a lower brain weight.

The ground-breaking research into Adverse Childhood Experiences (Felliti 1998) identified the link between childhood maltreatment and the long term implications on health and wellbeing. It started to investigate a high dropout rate at an obesity clinic only to find that obesity was linked to sexual abuse. The study has been replicated globally and has been pivotal in the realisation that those affected by neglectful, abusive and undesirable family circumstances go on to suffer with addiction, violence and unsocial behaviour and long-term chronic health conditions.

When working with the couple or pregnant mother, we will surely improve the impact of such trauma and the subsequent positive influence on the future wellbeing of the incoming soul. This starts with establishing a connection with the incoming soul.

I found it hard to believe that 50% of new mothers-to-be will not have a name prepared or form a bond with their baby until it's born "in case anything happens". Is this telling the baby they're not worth connecting with in case of separation or disappointment? That subconscious fear is palpable when assessing the relationship values in my sessions and breaks my heart to hear. So I offer connection to reassure them that they are welcome and loved no matter what the outcome. I accept the mother is doing her best with what she knows and encourage her to explore her relationship and improve bonding over our time together. The pregnancy takes on a whole new meaning when she connects. Babies know their parents' voices and clearly recognise those which are familiar to them, including ours as their maternity reflexologists.

Language and communication include non-verbal as well as oral skills. These reflect a tone and inflection which is interpreted and responded to accordingly. Listening to some mothers, they are really reluctant to name their babies, they use avoidance, limiting and fear driven terms and tones when referring to their fertility, pregnancy and birthing issues.

As a midwife I was well accustomed to the terms " failure to progress", "trial of labour" and now the attitude towards birthing brings its own wealth of terms that seek to coerce and disempower the birthing mother with a throw in of " you want a healthy baby don't you?", regardless of her personal perception of the situation. There is a rising movement of empowered birth workers supporting new mothers in creating an awakening and resurgence of innate feminine wisdom. Sisters are literally 'doing it for themselves', disengaging from the obstetric services, researching their options and birthing themselves in an endeavour of informed choice. Personally, I am loving this reclamation of the divine feminine, the creative force, admired in ancient civilisations and now rising again. There will always be a place for appropriate obstetric management in the event of emergencies and high-risk cases.

To watch a woman enter transition and go inward, rocking, connecting with her inner source, moaning in deeper tones to soothe her surges and pelvic pressure is magical and a privilege. No one taught her to do this. She is connecting with a greater consciousness, an inner knowing, connecting with all the mothers that went before her and the mothers in the divine matrix who will follow. You can see her energies changing in frequency with colours blending and moving as she transitions. Her vocalisations change as her resonant needs change. Orgasmic birthing really is a thing. In the right circumstances with oxytocin driven pleasure, feeling loved, safe and in control, the mother may climax as she births. So what if the birthing was as discrete and intimate as the creation as opposed to a floodlit performance with numerous strangers and fear driven protocols? Of course, I'm being dramatic to illustrate my point and which would you prefer? It's bad enough putting the light on when you need to pee in the middle of the night, half asleep let alone a rock concert and fireworks.

David Chamberlain's work demonstrated that when hypnotising mothers and children of 18 years of age the children were fully aware when they were told and regarded as going to be a "sickly child" or a "bad one". These remarks cause an imprint in the bio-field. Recall how you were called when you were young, the name your parents chose and the name you preferred. How did you feel when you were called 'bossy' or a chatterbox, a nuisance or naughty. These can conjure up frustration, anger and a feeling of being misunderstood even before we have verbal skills. Being treated differently by well-intentioned parents can create senses of injustice, rejection and jealousy too.

The beliefs we create in relation to our wellbeing, or dis-ease, creates inflammatory responses and there is a correlation to the types of diseases we develop according to the type of beliefs we make. Dis-ease is the embodiment of trauma. When we have a rigid outlook on life and are stuck in a bitter existence then our body will indeed represent such in the form of inflammatory, chronic cytokine storming and arthritic-like conditions and anything ending in 'itis'. The organs and systems affected can indicate the imbalances and we can often hear the causes in the words of those we are supporting. My work is facilitating others to transform their traumas and core beliefs to find and resolve the dis-ease processes and as a result, what was previously regarded as permanent deterioration and chronic illness subsides and pain reduces and is replaced with a new joie-de vivre. Think about what beliefs and terms we can hear our clients with fertility issues say: I don't have enough eggs; I'm too old; this is not good enough; I'm failing in that; I fear losing another pregnancy. By changing the words that we use again, we can create positive and encouraging change. How often have you caught yourself saying:" I can't", "won't", "mustn't", or "it's too difficult"; "my family is riddled with cancer so I'll get it"; when a change of thinking that "can", "will", "want" and that "I am healthy and happy" changes the emotion.

In every moment of every day of our current existence, our conscious mind is aware of only a millionth of what is actually going on. If we imagine watching a film on a huge cinema screen of 4000 million pixels, our conscious mind, what we are aware of will be a minuscule 4000 pixels, say the size of your fist; just think about that- a millionth of everything that is stimulating all our senses. 95-98 % of our day to day activity and thinking is automatic. This autoplay records and monitors our environment constantly, assessing for danger. If we experience something frightening or dangerous, our subconscious memory takes a 5D photograph, an imprint of everything; what is around us, within us, near us, the sounds, smells, tastes, and so much more. If we find ourselves in a similar situation and exposed to any of these factors, our protection mechanism via the amygdalae will race into action and we re-experience the reaction we had in the first place, unaware of the trigger. This may be how allergies and food sensitivities present and by reframing the original trauma the response is resolved and the sensitivity is dissipated, permanently. I've watched asthma resolve before my eyes. It's incredible what can be achieved, using modern energy psychology.

This, as you can see, is a massive subject and far too much to go into great detail here and I will discuss the origins of female reproductive cancer-related issues, beliefs and manifestations in Jane Sheehan's next book (The Gurus' Guide To Reflexology Book 3).

When we get it right

Becoming aware of how we get it wrong allows us to make waves to get it right. Trauma can be loved out of us. What a relief eh?

Neuroplasticy is the term for constant development of new neural pathways in our brains, 50,000 per second - as many stars as the 100 billion starred milky way - according to what we believe and perceive most about our environment, whether we are surviving or thriving and allows us to influence lasting change. It's fascinating to learn that every cell in our body is updated and changed approximately every 7 years. Just think, if we let go of our old shitty beliefs that hold us back, we can create a new perspective, a body that resonates the new mindset, leading to better health outcomes. How good will that feel? If we didn't create such self-sabotaging beliefs in the first place, would we perhaps have saved ourselves a lot of trouble and a whole load of unpleasant and heavy baggage along the way?

Wouldn't it be great if that couplings-to-be assessed their readiness to co-parent before the conception, in a state of preparedness as with any major life choice.   A holistic re-evaluation of priorities; connection and a making space for time to reconnect; disconnect from social media; co-create and raise the vibration of unconditional love and gratitude, far away from the current reality of the pressures of fearing failure at the first hurdle and facing anticipated fertility complications before the first temperature reading? Oh, and there's yet another app for that! Let's bring back the fun and joy to making babies in love.

When working with couples planning to conceive I ask them to consider an important question:
"If the incoming soul was waiting for the opportunity to come to you and looked down on your life at present what would they say? Why haven't they come yet?"

This approach has revealed some cracking insights into the lack of conception. Being too busy, distracted by commitments elsewhere, too stressful at work and even not having enough time or energy to have sex, have been realised. I've heard of one client who was so preoccupied with her fertility charts and planning she forgot to account for the fact that her partner worked off-shore for 2 weeks of the month. Coitus is rather essential for conception, wouldn't you agree? We need to create an opportunity, space and a warm welcome for them to come and fill.

The Swedish trial examining the sperm preferences in female follicular fluid showed "there is a growing appreciation that females can bias sperm use and paternity by exerting cryptic female choice for preferred males" in other words the female reproductive system influenced the choice of gametes that the ovum would bind with rather than another's sperm. I believe that the energetic connection between the partners presents a much deeper effect and this influences the choice and ability to procreate. When supporting clients with fertility issues we explore the relationship dynamics and have often found that once a relationship parts and a new more nourishing relationship commences, such fertility issues are no longer apparent. The connection was nonconductive to procreation. How many mothers are trying to substitute, fix or mend a dysfunctional relationship by having a baby?

In utero, the mother's maternal blood provides and supports the baby with 5HT (hydroxytriptamine), promoting brain development which has receptors in the central and peripheral nervous systems. These serotonin receptors modulate the release of neurotransmitters and hormones including GABA, epinephrin, and regulate oxytocin, prolactin and processes of appetite, aggression, cognition learning and memory among numerous others.

When the time is right and when left to Mother Nature, the incoming soul will initiate its birthing process. The macrophages that clean up the lungs of potential pathogens react to the production of surfactant protein A in the incoming soul's lungs, a fatty substance which lines the minuscule alveoli in preparation for inhalation and gaseous exchange once born, migrating to the uterus lining and triggering a chemical response which starts the birthing process. This can occur between 32 weeks and 42 weeks and may explain why some labours start later.

A birth remembered

The experiential learning that takes place during the process of birthing can be recalled long after the experience.

A friend recalls his time in utero:

"Strange as it sounds, I actually have faint memories of rebirth-swimming in the womb with a feeling of blissful weightlessness. And I was definitely aware of voices 'on the outside', particularly when my birth was in full flow.

I became conscious of being constricted; tight and unable to protect myself or make space with my armband, I believe that is why I've always, in my life outside, found enclosed spaces induce a mild sense of panic in me. (I once freaked out as child when I was caught under a bed in the same position.)

Lots of voices in what I guess must have been the later stages of birthing; and then the shock of the cold, and taking in air. Mild shock, I would imagine.

Back in 1959, I imagine my mother would have been made to lie on her back, which would have restricted my means of exit. And I can't help thinking it all could have been a more relaxed affair; less panic and noise. Hopefully next time it will be so. I was 14 days late by the way."

When asked, *"Do you procrastinate and need a deadline or rocket to get going?"*

His response was, *" Yes , usually. I'm a creative - full of self doubt. All my friends say they'll do anything to delay starting work. There are books on the subject- 'The War of Art' being one of them."*

The mode of delivery, I'd rather call it ' birthing', can create more beliefs. The compression of the head with forceps of another friend has created a self-protection strategy and a coping mechanism involving an aversion to anything metal towards her head. She still has a dent in her forehead to prove it. With a greater awareness in the role of biomechanics for birthing, acynclitism and malpresentation can be assisted into better realignment with improved outcomes. This can only be good news.

The golden hour after birth is a precious primordial time where the 9 step process to the first feed must be honoured. When interrupted, the first feed and latch will be delayed and the opportunity for bonding may lose its efficacy. This stepped process includes the initial cry after emergence, an awake time calmly looking for mother's face and listening, crawling up the mother's body initiating the cross body reflex development and cerebral connection of the corpus collosum, the bridge between the left and right hemispheres. Those who are bum shufflers and don't crawl may be more likely to experience developmental delays. Babies need to crawl. Cultures whose children are carried and do not set foot on the ground for the first year become great followers of protocols but not necessarily great problem solvers or planners.

Synthetic oxytocin used to induce and augment labour, has been shown to affect the oxytocin receptors and the subsequent sensitivity of the uterus to the mother's own natural oxytocin, reducing perfusion of the placenta, causing fatal distress; affecting the mother's enjoyment of the process, bonding and timing of the first feed. (SW)

We've all heard of women trying anything to get things going and maybe you've been asked to induce labour with your magic hands? While induction and any reference to or notion that reflexology can be used, starting things off must be avoided if we are to maintain a mindset of support and resist the connotation that we can make such a prescriptive and medical decision to end the pregnancy. We are better equipped to facilitate a supportive narrative encouraging the mother to enjoy the last few weeks and days, knowing that all her baby's needs are being met effortlessly and cherish this time for herself. I'm concerned for the practitioners' requests for 'those acupressure points to fiddle with to get her started' posts when the basic fundaments of her needs can be met and accomplished using a multilevel approach to the Endocrine Balancing. Even medical inductions are unsuccessful when the pregnancy is not fully mature, starting a cascade of intervention.

Steven Porges' work with his Polyvagal Theory explores the relation of the three unique branches of the part of our autonomic nervous system that controls our involuntary functions like heart beating and breathing, the 10th cranial nerve, the 'wandering' vagus nerve, which controls specific parts of our body and affects the relative function according to our perceptions of safety or threat within our environment. By working with an understanding of how our bodies react to trauma enables us to support a recovery and resolution.

Interestingly the smile and facial expressions of a baby creates an oxytocin-fired boost to mum's brain and is reciprocated when mum responds to baby's expressions. Research showed the devastating impact that a fixed facial expression of the mother caused resulting in separation anxiety. My concerns widen to the impact of the mandatory mask-wearing currently required. So much expression is expressed with subtle almost imperceptible mannerisms in the face which can, if the practitioner is unaware, trigger abreactions in traumatised individuals. Try it with a friend and ask them to tut and roll their eyes at a remark you make. Where do you feel it?

Is it any wonder that skin conditions like eczema and psoriasis present with an underlying belief of separation and loss of connection? This, I believe, is compounded when artificial substitutes are given. Imagine the separation of the mother cow constantly impregnated and the calf removed to maintain her milk supply. They grieve for weeks. That resonance will trigger that in us. Asthma is the adaptive phase of an allergen response. Later chronic inflammatory issues including arthritis may develop. Lung and breathing issues can be related to feeling of overwhelm and suffocation, grief and bereavement. We are what we eat so please choose wisely. When using Emotional Freedom Technique for eczema on the baby, working with mum's anxiety first can often resolve the transferred trauma and subsequent symptoms. It makes so much sense when searching for core beliefs.

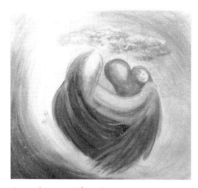

A mother's grief in the vortex, painting by Jennifer Tribe ©

A Dutch study examining the effects on the adult off-spring of mothers exposed to a Dutch famine during preconception and pregnancy in 1944-45 showed an increase in depression and poorer health outcomes. Adult children of Holocaust survivors experiencing PTSD, experienced poorer long-term health outcomes, and unhealthy behaviours. This demonstrates inherited trauma, an imprint on the cellular memory of the unborn and yet to be conceived, of those experiencing PTSD.

When we consider that when our grandmother was pregnant with our mother she possessed all her primordial cells in her ovaries, one of which became you. Any trauma our grandmothers experienced may well have been recorded in our biofield and led to behaviour pattern accordingly. I've worked with past lives and worked remotely, and surrogately too with fascinating results.

We think we have time

Time is an illusion. Time is not a linear line with a beginning or end. When teaching, I ask my students to draw two dots on the ends of an A4 piece of paper: a beginning and an end, a timeline. Then I ask them to connect the dots. They always draw a straight line. I then screw my piece of paper up and twist it so the dots touch.

The beginning and end run simultaneously with the now. The creases in the paper represent experiences, trials and empirical experiences along the way.

I will describe the "Infinity Sweep" I teach to clear an energetic field in my section on 'How we can support the incoming soul'.

Recognising our personal birthing story

In order to become an effective reflexology practitioner in this field of expertise, we must consider our own experiences, our own journey. None of us are perfect but rather perfectly imperfect; imperfectly perfect. The unique insight into our personal development from an early age, is not one to immerse in distress but the joy of unraveling the wonder of where those self-sabotaging beliefs came from. Like an acorn with the potential to generate a dark foreboding forest; one flawed misconception may give rise to a lifetime of feeling unworthy of happy experiences and joyful abundance, settling for suboptimal, violent relationships, addiction, self-harm and abuse.

The relief is, that we can rewrite the past, change the script. By replanting the acorn in new soil, that forest can become the most enchanted wood leading to a gloriously sunny meadow filled with flowers and life. What would you choose?

I know of many therapists whose life-long ambition is personal development to enable them to be their best in their professional capacity, helping and supporting others. Unfortunately there are as many, fearfully avoiding the opportunity for discovery, only to continue perhaps in denial of any need to face the past or consider their current standing as a wounded warrior, unaware that their very intentions will be affected by the very resonance of such vibrational baggage.

It takes great courage to contemplate change from our comfort zones and the familiarity of our old ways of thinking. This is why I am excited to offer such opportunities by way of transformational retreats for therapists, midwives and other health care professionals. If we are to start with ourselves and show by example, the effect will be exponential in these challenging times. My plan is not to retrigger unpleasant memories or trawl through disassociated childhood traumas to be awake to the endless possibilities of the power achieved when letting go of what we think we need to keep to identify with.

Imagine the freedom of just being in the present moment with no concerns and worries and excited in anticipation of what's to happen next. Imagine feeling ready to be reborn in the current moment, a slate wiped clean of all wrong doings by you and done to you or because of you.

So what if I told you that we choose our mothers and that our children chose us to mother them? Crazy?

This leads me onto another dear friend who relayed her story of not wanting to find herself pregnant with her second child nine months after the birth of her first, after forced relations. She felt guilty about feeling that her time with her first daughter would now be cramped with the new sibling-to-be, having struggled to conceive her for 4 years.

Several years later, having read Christine Northrup's book " Mothers and daughters", something resonated deeply inside her and she wrote down her thoughts on two scraps of paper. Further years followed and she showed the remnants to her second daughter who immediately understood what her mother had realised. She had chosen her mum and had come to teach her about love and while they had time together as her older sibling was at university, their bond became even closer.

Now consider how we can prepare ourselves to support the next generation with a wiser and more open heart and mind.

So how can we support the incoming souls with reflexology?

Having considered and perhaps reframed our own experiences and forgiven ourselves for doing our best with the resources available to us at the time, we are more open to offering a vibration resonant with unconditional love, a frequency of 555Hz., (There are many meditations and videos of binaural beats of various frequencies and properties to listen to on media channels), a warm soft pink colour for those who are visual therapists. This sets the tone for the session and when in doubt, consider ourselves as the prism refracting the pure

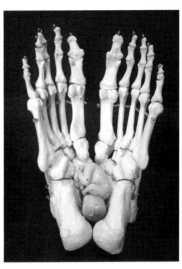

Pregnancy on the feet, with permission Maternity Reflexology Consortium ©

vibrational white light in all its glorious fractals. When regarding the question of protection, I ask "from what?". If we consider we need protection from dark energies, entities and the like, perhaps we are attracting to us a vibration which resonates with what we are desiring protection from by just thinking about it. Thought creates emotion and moves energy. My suggestion is to move your focus to one of outshining the darkness. We all have a pilot light near our heart from which source consciousness radiates. What could be simpler than turning it up? Make it brighter and brighter. This is so simple, it's child's play. Work with love, not fear and if you sense you are self-checking and find you need to adjust your settings, do so.

Our pineal grand is our solar light information receptor and formerly much larger in size. This incredible structure recognised in ancient civilisations and regarded as the all-seeing eye, (the eye of Horus in Egyptian teachings) contains retinal cells and is the driver of our circadian rhythms and also known as our 'third eye'. The solar, holonomic and geometric frequencies are absorbed and downloaded, interpreted and transformed into our hormonal messengers of the endocrine system.

In the developing embryo, heart cells develop and start beating prior to the development of the brain; yes, we are heart-led not brain-led. Follow your heart , not your head. If somethings feels innately right - or wrong, for that matter, you will feel it in your heart and solar plexus, (our gut instinct shows that we have a brain there too).

When we are in alignment our body feels energised, in tune, connected, effortless, and feels light and in love with life. As the toroidal forces flow round and through our heart-field, what we feel in our hearts will influence that which we magnetise to use. Do you remember sprinkling iron filings over magnets at school? Our hearts are 500 times more magnetic than our brain. We, therefore, can attract more with our heart than our brain. Ever felt fearful of a lack of finances only to find three appliances fail within a few days, or gain a parking ticket or a speeding fine?

For a greater understanding of the sacred geometric properties of our light body matrix I suggest you check out the following link and explore the fascinating free videos provided by TheTemplate.org at http://bit.ly/TemplateClearandProtect ›

Here you will be enlightened to discover how long we have been suppressed and coerced into believing we are so much less than we really are, plus an array of information.

When working with the Endocrine Balancing we include the placenta in the non-pregnant uterine reflex zone. The placenta is regarded as a unique chakra recording the emotional journey of the incoming soul's passage earthside. Many make up products contain placental tissue and facial treatment products contain tissues from newborns' foreskins for their rejuvenating youth preserving properties. These alarming revelations may be exacerbated when we realise that any trauma sustained, particularly during circumcision, may be still resonating in the cellular memory in those applications.

Sound therapy has a valuable place in recalibrating trauma. Ever listened to live music or the song from childhood and been moved to tears? (Jackie and 'Snowy white horses' for me.) Heard the infectious giggling of an infant and couldn't resist laughing yourself? That's what I call contagious plus a health benefit.

Getting into the vortex

When I prepare for our sessions I find that self-regulation of my own emotional state using HeartMath (breathe in for 6, out for 6, through the heart), which improves the coherence of our brainwaves to the heart field. With practice, it really helps me achieve relaxation swiftly. Handy when something untoward happens in the final moments before they arrive on your doorstep.

As with any ceremony, I like to consider all my senses. Incense, and pregnancy safe aromatherapy blends create an ambience while palo santo and white sage sprays give an alternative to smoking the room. If you like crystals then rose quartz , moonstone and smokey quartz are very grounding, though moon stone can be too strong to wear around the full moon, I'm told.

If you are a practitioner that is working from home and finds it difficult to separate your work/life balance then a uniform or work clothes help enormously. I know this may feel basic and common sense but reflect on the colours you wear too. Black is very absorbing and white radiating. If. for example, the client's sacral chakra area is a focus for libido and fertility work then orange lingerie may be in order. Failing that, a coloured shawl around the area works well too.

When in doubt, white covers all bases. Intention is key.

Washing my hands before beginning allows me time to appreciate the feeling of the flow and cleansing of the energy passing through my hands and around my field.

Especially mindful when working with newly pregnant clients and those preparing to conceive, I like to ask permission to proceed, handing the power and consent over to the mother. This changes the whole intention. We are not working to fix anything but to support the rebalancing of traumatic imprints. When supporting medicated fertility protocols then we need to be aware of the intentions of the medication in order to support their action effectively. We don't wish the medication to metabolise too rapidly or encourage egg release prior to harvesting so I suggest we decline a 48 hour window prior to collection. We can reconvene straight after gamete and donor implantation in an effort to support the endometrial enveloping the new blastocyst.

Contraindications to consider when working with incoming souls include when we don't feel we have the confidence to proceed or a gut feeling to delay or avoid treating that we need to honour. The others include the usual red flags and DVT if not being treated.

Keep an open mind and allow your conscious mind to relax into your treatment and let go of the idea of the 'routine' which provides a safe starting block for a strong foundation to your practice. Now I encourage you to go with the flow more and let your intuition guide you. Ask yourself:" what am I meant to now see and hear and feel?' I've witnessed the indigo bubbles of prephysical consciousness hovering around the medial pelvic area a week before conception. I knew with certainty what I was seeing and the words "a baby's coming" poured from my mouth. Fortunately, this was music to the mum-to-be's ears as she had just stopped the pill to plan her family. I have a well-established pre-blurb filter in place now, have you?

When assessing the spine, be aware of any areas of tension and imbalance and these may correspond to the imprint of the conception journey to birth similar to the mapping of the 'Prenatal Pattern' in the Metamorphic Technique. Neck issues may be related to beliefs surrounding injustice and uncertainty and the neck area on the spine on the medial side of the heel corresponds to conception time. So, ask the client whether they were aware of any concerns or challenges around their conception? This may have never been discussed and sows the seeds for contemplation during the rest of the session. Many will then come forward with some indication when they have relaxed and their subconscious mind has released some information. Thus the pelvic area corresponds to birthing and this is no surprise here, when we consider the birthing of a new baby is also the birthing of a new mother as she taps into her own birthing experience as she moves, moans and traverses dimensions connecting to her higher self.

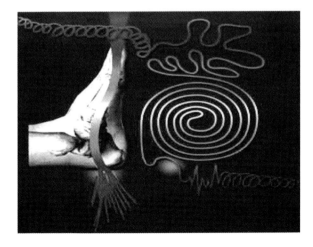

Metaphysical Birth Picture of the foot, with permission The Maternity Reflexology Consortium ©

We are so privileged to work with the new-born souls and I only compliment the beautiful babies. They will grow up seeking reassurance and constant approval to explore and, if distracted by mobile devices and lack of facial recognition and acknowledgement, their brains will not develop properly. This was shown in those of children 'raised' in Romanian orphanages where the telomeres, (caps on DNA strands related to ageing), were found to be shorter in children with poorer health outcomes. Without love, the brain disengages and we die from disconnection. (Sue Gerhardt)

The creation of the 'Infinity Sweep'

While working with clients in my transformation work, it became apparent that I needed a technique that would assist a change, a mopping up and clearing out technique and I pondered a while. This happened during a virtual session and then it came to me. I asked the client to visualise going back to their first experience of life in whatever shape of form that came up and to bring all the unhelpful shit (a great word that describes all unhelpful baggage) from the beginning of time and compress it into a really dense black hole and bring it to now. Then by compressing it into the most beautiful diamond, it would become the dazzling, sustaining power that drives all hope dreams and ambition for the future and to take it to the farthest point of existence and then bring it back to the present moment.

This, simply applied to reflexology, is to work in figures of 8 (the power number, the symbol of infinity) over any areas requiring adjustment in order to re-establish a harmonic resonance of balance. The fluidity of the movement becomes like a pendulum, being and flowing, a slightly different angle the next time and a continuum of connection.

Use it over the reflex zones, over the endocrine organs and the incoming soul in the pregnant feet and in the special interdimensional zone between the feet. Use off body light touch first before progressing to use increasing layers of pressure. We are not only working physically but with all aspects of the energetic body.

Try it on yourself first. It is incredibly effective and mind-blowingly simple. Child's play. Teach children how to soothe bruising and bumps with it. Support each other in the family.

I look forward to your feedback.

Summary

I would like to summarise by suggesting that we all need to support change NOW, in order to welcome the incoming souls into a global consciousness of infinite love and gratitude.

To play our part we must look into our own hearts and recognise that WE are our starting point.

It is never too late to start and when we are ready to challenge our perspectives learned from our own experiences and the beliefs of those who influenced our upbringing, miracles happen. We chose them after all. What are we here for?

When we forgive ourselves and those who we feel have hurt us, we release the shackles of what no longer serves us, creating an openness to previously unimagineable possibilities.

Just as an innocent child sees the world, so we see the greater potential around us and recognise those resonating on the same path to a kinder, more loving utopia for us all.

We are not here to fix but to create and experience all aspects of love in all her guises and the path is not necessarily an easy one to endure and may perhaps become a more rewarding journey because of it.

The incoming souls will enter our divine matrix with a greater consciousness that we will have facilitated by our learning and expansion. They will show us a better way to be.

To live in constant questioning brings an energetic boost to our quantum reality and when asking "how does it get any better than this and what else is possible?" will attract an unfolding like we've never experienced before.

We are who we've been waiting for.

Trust that our best is good enough and the more we experience the more our best evolves.

We are the universe.

About Jennifer (Jenni) Tribe

Jenni works with those wishing to make peace with the past, find passion and purpose and create a life to love. She has a special interest in all things associated with pregnancy, lack and loss and a loss of self-worth.

A former Nurse and Midwife of 30 years' experience, disillusioned with the medical models designed to treat chronic health issues without addressing the root cause, took a leap of faith in order to support others, after overcoming her own severe perinatal, postnatal and perimenopausal mental health challenges following bereavement and pregnancy-loss.

Mother, motivational speaker, writer, nature-lover, wild swimmer, author-to-be, procrastinator, perfectionist, maternity reflexology trainer, transformation retreats organiser,

Energy psychology practitioner, EFT trainer, NLP Coach, Hypnosis, Timeline TherapyTM practitioner, Matrix and Birth Re-imprinting practitioner, Life Purpose, Founding member of The Maternity Reflexology Consortium, Association of Radical Midwives member ARM, Association of Prenatal and Perinatal Psychology and Health APPPAH, Full member Association of Reflexologists

JenniTribe.com
TheTransformationTribe.uk
Maternity-Reflexology.co.uk

Menopause
by Jane Sheehan
(from Norwich)

Menopause
by Jane Sheehan (from Norwich)

(Before I talk about menopause, I would just like to say that I am NOT the Footreader! I am the other Jane Sheehan. We often get mistaken for each other and people are often confused especially when we sat next to each other at the FHT Awards ceremony where we were both nominated. I was referred to as 'Jane Sheehan from Norwich')

Menopause in our society is often seen as something to be feared and endured or at least as a great inconvenience. It is generally not something to be welcomed, embraced or seen in a positive light. The same could be said of the onset of menstruation.

By contrast, in some societies both of these stages in a woman's life are celebrated with joy and are marked by beautiful ceremonies to honour the change and the transition into a new phase of life. Change is as inevitable as night following day and yet is often something we resist with all our might. This makes the process more challenging than it need be and developing an ability to 'go with the flow' can be extremely helpful.

Some women feel that their bodies are failing them, that this is the beginning of the end. In reality though, after menopause women may have 30 or 40 more years to live. So rather than an end instead it can be seen as a time to pause and to look for ways that will help us to cherish ourselves as we move into our wisest years with improved health and more of a feeling of being comfortable in our skins.

The menopause usually occurs between the ages of 40 and 58 – the average age being 51years. It is the natural end of a woman's menstrual cycle and is usually formally recognised as being 12 months after the final period.

However, the perimenopause (meaning 'around menopause') begins earlier, as the balance of hormones begins to shift, and some symptoms may continue beyond the cessation of periods for several months or years. The oestrogen which has been produced by the ovaries gradually decreases, and the adrenal glands start to make oestrogen and androgen to replace this. In a healthy woman this whole natural process can be smooth and easy, but many women do not find the transition easy and may experience troublesome symptoms including:

- Hot flushes/night sweats
- Insomnia/palpitations
- Headaches/poor memory
- Anxiety/Depression
- Weight gain
- Irritability/mood swings
- Joint pain/stiffness
- Reduced libido/vaginal dryness
- Fatigue
- Urinary frequency/leakage

The perimenopause

During perimenopause, the menstrual cycles may change, with bleeds becoming heavier, lighter, closer together or further apart, or any combination of these, due to the decline in ovarian function. This can cause feelings of being out of control and heralds the first signs of the tide of change. We may feel more irritable than usual with circumstances that, prior to this have been manageable. For example, we may feel that we no longer want to be the person that everyone relies upon, whether at home or work or with any areas of unresolved stress.

The hormones which have played a huge part in enabling us to bring up our children and nurture our families (and have done so to ensure that we reproduce and continue as a species) are now changing. As our childbearing years are coming to a close it is as though we are being 'returned to ourselves' without that layer of hormones dictating our moods etc. It is no coincidence that this often happens around the time when children have grown up and leave home - the 'empty nest'. Women may find they no longer want to do the job they have done for many years or they may start to wonder what they want for themselves for rest of their lives.

Research has shown that not only are the levels of hormones in the body changing, but there are other changes taking place in the nervous system. These have the effect of the circuits in the brain being 'rewired', so this is an important developmental stage in a woman's life.

Levels of oestrogen and progesterone affect the limbic area and the temporal lobe of the brain and, as in the second half of your cycle, it may be more difficult to ignore unresolved stressors, so this is the same during the perimenopause. This may be seen as 'a problem with your hormones' but is in fact your inner wisdom trying to get your attention and you may find it difficult to focus or to remember things. During the first half of your menstrual cycle the rising oestrogen levels make it easier to overlook things in order to carry on with what you are doing in your life. When the levels fluctuate and then fall at menopause it is then much more difficult to overlook things that you are not happy with in your life.

Listening to your inner wisdom becomes even more important at this time than possibly ever before. As the levels of FSH and LH increase and then level out at menopause this enables us to have a constant flow of connection with our own inner wisdom, rather than the ebb and flow which tends to happen during the menstrual cycle.

It seems that when a woman fights against the natural process of change and wants everything to remain as it always has been, she will tend to experience more difficulties at this time. The key is for her to really 'listen' to herself, to her body and her inner knowing, so she can embrace the next phase of her life as a woman of wisdom.

The menopause is often seen as the end of youth and the ability to give birth to new life. However, it can be looked on as a gift, as an opportunity for a woman to reconnect with her intuition and to embark upon a new phase of life which she is creating, a time to cherish herself. As the song says, "I am what I am, I am my own special creation". What an adventure this could be!

Reflexology and the menopause

A woman will be receiving a variety of different sorts of information from many directions about her menopause. There are no right and wrong ways of dealing with it and the important thing is that your client is making the informed choices that work best for her. She may decide to take HRT (hormone replacement therapy) or she may be looking at going down a more natural route, including complementary therapy in her self-care.

As discussed, the symptoms that your client may be experiencing stem from the fluctuating hormone levels. For example, as the levels of oestrogen and progesterone drop during perimenopause, the buffer effect that they have against cortisol is diminished and increased cortisol levels are associated with anxiety.

The usual advice for lowering cortisol levels is to find ways of managing stress effectively doing things such as exercise, meditation, yoga, tai chi, activities that you enjoy – and of course, reflexology.

Reflexology is a very useful support at this time as it is a fabulous treatment for reducing stress. When I first trained in 2000, my teacher said that if all that reflexology did was to reduce stress, then that would be enough.

Reflexology helps your clients to sink into a deep relaxation and has been shown to significantly reduce stress and anxiety; clients experience increased feelings of ease and wellbeing.

Reflexology may also help improve mood, release tension and aid sleep, which helps to ease stresses being experienced during this transitional time and helps us to cope more easily.

Chinese medicine and the menopause

When I worked with patients in a Palliative Care Unit, I was treating a young woman who was experiencing severe and distressing hot flushes as a result of her medications. Reflexology sessions didn't seem to be helping with this symptom.

My Shiatsu training included the study of Chinese medicine and the use of acupressure points, so I decided to incorporate some points which would have a chance of helping. The young woman came for fortnightly appointments and she was overjoyed to find that her hot flushes reduced to a manageable level! She found that the effects lasted just under 2 weeks, and the day before she came for her next treatment the flushes would have returned.

Since that time there are a few points that I will always include in treatments for a woman who is navigating the menopause. I find this greatly enhances the treatment and I recommend incorporating them into your reflexology sessions – particularly to address hot flushes. I also draw on other advice to support her, using the valuable perspective of Chinese medicine.

Chinese medicine is a huge field of study, with roots going back over 5,000 years, so I will only touch on it very lightly here, to show how we can draw on some simple but powerful tools from this tradition to aid us in supporting women through the menopause.

In Chinese cosmology everything in the universe is considered to be made up of **Qi**. This is often described as energy but in the widest sense it also encompasses matter – as in Einstein's famous equation $E=MC2$. The Chinese character for Qi includes both uncooked rice and steam, representing the continuum of energy and matter.

The human body is viewed as a vortex of energy and other 'Vital Substances' interacting with each other to form an organism. The basis of all is Qi and the other Substances are manifestations of Qi varying from the physical to the spiritual (note the western body/mind duality does not exist in this system).

The body's Qi has 3 sources: 'Source Qi', from both our parents; 'Earth Qi', from the food and fluids we ingest; 'Heavens Qi', from the breath.

Qi flows around the body in a network of channels known as meridians – along which the acupressure points are located. When we press a point, we activate the Qi in the meridian and we're able to connect with our receivers on all levels, from the physical to the spiritual. Meridian theory forms the basis for some schools of reflexology, so will be familiar to some of you already.

The Chinese understanding of health is based on a balance of Yin and Yang in the body/mind. Yin and Yang are opposite yet interdependent polarities which are only ever relative to one another.

The Yin principle is cooling, nourishing, moistening, relaxing

The Yang principle is warming, activating, transforming, moving

In Chinese medicine each meridian is connected to an 'Organ' and it's important to know that these Organs are not the same as their western medical equivalents – we use capital letters (e.g. Kidney / Liver) to differentiate them. They have many associations on every level, including the physical, emotional, psychological and spiritual levels and each has a range of different functions in the human metabolism.

The Kidneys underpin all metabolic activity and are known as the foundation of Yin and Yang in the body. They store the Source Qi, which is Yang in nature and fuels all activity. They also store another Vital Substance known as **Essence**, which is Yin in nature and forms the basis for the physical substance of the body. Both these Yin and Yang aspects are received from our parents at the moment of conception and are equivalent to our 'genetic package'. Our basic constitution, strength and stamina are associated with the Kidneys and they govern birth, growth, reproduction, and development through the stages of life.

I describe the Kidneys to my clients as being the 'batteries of the body'. Kidney Qi naturally diminishes with age and is particularly depleted by overwork, long term stress and by sexual activity for men and childbearing for women. The Kidneys benefit most from a balance between activity and rest, a healthy diet, breathing exercises and a moderate lifestyle.

The gateways of change

Chinese medicine sees the menopause as one of the 'Gateways of Change' in a woman's life. These gateways are certain times in our lives when we are in transition from one phase of life to the next. They are times when there is powerful hormonal and emotional activity taking place and significant change is occurring:

- Birth and perinatal period
- Puberty
- Onset of sexual activity
- Pregnancy and childbirth
- Menopause

These are particular times when our whole constitution can be strengthened or weakened so we need to take extra care of ourselves. We may be more susceptible to dis-ease but likewise, we may experience better health if we maintain a healthy and balanced lifestyle. This involves avoiding undue emotional stress and tension, working too hard, and any extremes.

From the energetic perspective of Chinese medicine then, the basis of many of the difficulties which women may experience during menopause stems from the natural decline of the Kidney energy with age. Menopausal symptoms in particular tend to reflect Deficiency of Kidney Yin, the classic signs of which include: fatigue, restlessness, insomnia, feeling hot and night sweats. Interestingly osteoporosis is also a sign of Kidney Yin Deficiency in Chinese medicine terms.

However, the natural decline of Kidney energy as we age is ideally balanced with the increase of its traditional 'Virtue' which is Wisdom!

Other Organs which have specific roles in relation to the female reproductive system and the menstrual cycle are the **Spleen and Liver** and I will also include reference to a few important points on those meridians, which can help to rebalance, replenish and support the whole system.

As well as Qi and Essence, other Vital Substances relevant for us to know a little about are **Blood and Shen.** Blood in Chinese medicine is more than the red fluid in our cardio-vascular system, it is more like the Yin equivalent to Qi. Being Yin, it has those 'cooling, nourishing, moistening and relaxing' qualities. On a psychological level it is also about feeling at ease and about 'how kind we can be to ourselves'. When we are Blood Deficient, symptoms may include: dry skin, dry hair, irritability and depression, insomnia (especially trouble getting off to sleep), poor memory, dizziness, restlessness and fatigue.

The Shen is often translated as Spirit and is linked both to our Higher Self and to our sense of self in this world. It is also associated with the mind, with the ability to form thoughts, think clearly and to be fully present with our awareness. In Chinese medicine there are many practices to cultivate a quiet mind, which is associated with longevity and wellbeing.

Chinese medicine is very complex, but these are the bare bones of where the menopause fits in to its landscape.

How to incorporate acupressure points into your treatment

Apply gentle perpendicular pressure to the point. Breathe and really relax yourself as you press. Remember these are 'energetic points' so you do not have to press them hard. You are connecting into a whole energetic system of body/mind/spirit. It is as though you are plugging in to the inner wisdom of their body, lighting up the meridian network and encouraging it to activate and find its balance wherever it is most needed. Intention is an important element here so focus on what you are aiming to achieve to enhance the process, for example 'calming the Mind' or 'nourishing the Yin'. Try this on yourself. You will find that you can connect deeply but that it feels completely different to just pressing.

How to help your reflexology client

For all your clients I am assuming that you will give a full whole person reflexology treatment including an endocrine balance of your choice.

In addition to that, I am suggesting some areas where you may like to focus extra attention. Following this are specific acupressure points, some single and some in combination, to enhance your treatments. Each point has many different 'actions' and I am just including a few of the most relevant here. Note: The drawings that relate to these points (figures 1 to 9) are shown on pages 239 and 240.

1   Hot flushes

If your client is experiencing hot flushes the relaxation element of reflexology will be very important. If you remember, in Chinese medicine the client will have Kidney Yin Deficiency and will need rest and relaxation to nourish the Kidneys.

Besides your whole-body reflexology treatment, areas to give extra attention to will be:

- The Endocrine system to balance hormonal activity
- Pituitary to promote endocrine balance
- Solar plexus to calm and relax to alleviate stress
- Kidney 1, 3, 6, 7, and Liver 3 <Fig 4, 1,2,3, 5>

Acupressure points
Kidney 3 (Figure 1)
Actions:
- Tonifies the Kidney
- Benefits Essence
- Nourishes Yin and Clears Heat
- Benefits the uterus

Kidney 7 (Figure 2)
Actions:
- Tonifies the Kidney
- Regulates sweating

Kidney 6 (Figure 3)

Actions:

- Nourishes Yin
- Clears Heat
- Cools the Blood
- Calms the Spirit

Apply perpendicular pressure to each of these points in turn and then apply a linking technique holding all three points at the same time. Always ensure your hand is in a comfortable relaxed position and when linking points, just hold gently and focus your intention in your mind.

The heat experienced by women having hot flushes and night sweats is known as Deficient or Empty Heat in Chinese Medicine. I explain this to clients by describing the pictogram representing Qi. This is of a fire with a pot of rice boiling above it, and the steam that rises off this is Qi. If the pan boils dry the rice would then start to burn and there would be no steam. This situation is Empty Heat as the problem is not an excess of heat but rather insufficient water in the pot. In the same way, the hot flushes are happening because there is not enough Yin, which most of all needs rest to replenish it.

Kidney 1 (Figure 4)
Actions:

- Tonifies Yin
- Clears Heat
- Calms the mind – calming anxiety

Combine Kidney 1 with Liver 3 for hot flushes, it will draw Qi down from the head and upper body. Hold both points simultaneously. Liver 3 is a strong point and can be sensitive.

Liver 3 (Figure 4)

Actions:

- Promotes the Smooth Flow of Liver Qi
- Calms the Shen (Spirit/Mind)
- Nourishes Liver Yin and Liver Blood
- Regulates Menstruation

Self-help

For women experiencing hot flushes, **rest** is the single most important element for recovery, mentally and physically. To replenish Kidney Qi you really need to lie down, sitting doesn't really do it.

- Hot flushes will occur more during stressful situations, so reduce stress wherever possible.
- Avoid excessive exercise – switch to gentle relaxing exercise such as Qigong, Tai Chi, Yoga or walking, ideally in nature.
- Avoid late nights.
- A good self-help yoga pose: lying down with legs fully supported by a wall. Direct your client to lie on their side and shuffle their buttocks right up to the wall, then turn onto their back. In this way the legs will be fully supported.
- Relaxation MP3s can be useful as they give a little oasis of calm in the day, even for 5 minutes a couple of times a day.

Dietary advice

Try to avoid or reduce stimulants such as coffee, caffeine, alcohol, tobacco, refined and processed food and excessive salt.

Chinese medicine views food from a different perspective and focuses on its energetic effects. Some specifically 'cooling' foods include spinach, celery and cucumber - in fact, salad vegetables generally tend to have cooling energy as do most fresh fruits. Wheatgerm tonifies the Yin, whole wheat is said to 'Calm the Spirit'.

2 Insomnia

Insomnia may lead to feelings of tiredness, worry and fearfulness (Fear is the emotion which is associated with the Kidney energy system).

Besides your whole-body reflexology treatment, areas to give extra attention to will be:

- Diaphragm - to help deeper breathing and relaxation
- Solar plexus - to relieve anxiety and help relaxation
- Spine and spinal nerves - to ease tension, balance and calm the nervous system
- Head, neck and shoulders - to ease tension and help relaxation
- Vagus nerve - to stimulate the release of oxytocin which promotes relaxation, a sense of wellbeing and improved digestion.
- Adrenal glands - hold points or gently stroke in a downward movement to calm the production of adrenalin
- Lung and chest area - to help deeper breathing and promote relaxation
- Kidney 1 (see above)

Acupressure points
Kidney 1
- Calms the Mind - reducing anxiety, improving relaxation and enabling sleep *(Figure 4)*

3 Headaches

Besides your whole-body reflexology treatment, areas to give extra attention to will be:
- Head/neck and sinus reflexes - to relieve tension held in these areas and to improve blood flow to area

- Solar plexus - to help relaxation and achieve a calm feeling. Hold solar plexus reflex and if it feels appropriate, allow your thumb to softly sink into it
- Liver reflex - to cleanse and detoxify. In Chinese medicine the Liver is associated with the emotions of frustration and anger, and with thought processes, so you will be working on multiple levels, physical, mental and emotional
- Spine and spinal nerves - your aim is to soothe the nervous system
- Liver 3 *(Figure 5)*
- Kidney 1 with Liver 3 (see above) *(Figures 4 and 5)*
- Large Intestine 4 *(Figure 6)*

Acupressure points

Liver 3

- Promotes the smooth flow of Qi around the body *(Figure 5)*

Very useful for headaches and migraines. Hold the points on both feet simultaneously and visualise drawing energy down the body

Kidney 1 & Liver 3

This is a good combination to hold simultaneously for relieving headaches. *(Figures 4 and 5)*

Large Intestine 4

Between the 1st and 2nd metacarpal bones, approximately in the middle of the second bone on the radial side. Apply perpendicular pressure horizontally – towards the ulna side of the hand *(Figure 6)*

Actions:
- Relieves pain
- NB Induces labour so is contra-indicated during pregnancy

Self-help

Show your client how to hold the relaxing solar plexus point in the centre of the palm of the hand. This is also a significant acupressure point for calming the mind.

Dietary advice

Avoid heating stimulants such as coffee, sugar, alcohol. Yin boosting foods include wheatgerm and mung beans.

4 Anxiety

Besides your whole-body reflexology treatment, areas to give extra attention to will be:

- Solar plexus - to promote deep relaxation
- Adrenal glands - to calm the effects of the fight/ flight response
- Respiratory system - to regulate breathing to promote calmness throughout the mind and body
- Nervous system - to balance the sympathetic and parasympathetic nervous system
- Spleen 6 *(Figure 6)*
- Heart Protector 6 *(Figure 8)*

Acupressure Points

Spleen 6

4 finger widths directly above the tip of the medial malleolus on the posterior border of the tibia. *(Figure 7)*

Actions:
- Calms the Mind
- Strengthens the Spleen

- Nourishes Blood and Yin
- Helps reproductive system issues
- Assists irregular menstruation
- Contraindicated in pregnancy

The Spleen is associated with the Earth Element in Chinese medicine and, as well as being linked to the female reproductive system, is also to do with feeling grounded and supported. It is also associated with 'worry and overthinking' and several points on the Spleen meridian are used specifically to calm the Mind. When someone is anxious, they are likely to be feeling ungrounded, so strengthening the Spleen energy and calming the Mind can both be beneficial.

Heart Protector 6

(Figure 8) 3 fingers widths proximal to the transverse wrist crease (with palm facing up) between the tendons of palmaris longus and flexor carpi radialis.

Actions:
- Regulates Heart Qi
- Calms the Mind
- Helps agitation, restlessness & insomnia

The Heart Protector meridian is associated with the Fire Element. This Element is affected by excessive emotion and when out of balance it can result in anxiety. When balanced there is a feeling of calm.

Self-help

Deep abdominal breathing is very calming and good for nourishing the Yin. When you slow down the exhalation you are connecting with the parasympathetic nervous system which automatically initiates the relaxation response.

There are many Apps for meditation and Mindfulness which can be useful. Deep relaxations and Yoga Nidras are also available on the internet. It is worth trying a few as it is important that your client finds the person's voice easy to listen to.

You can show your client how to find Heart Protector 6 to use if feelings of anxiety are starting.

Show your client how to use the Solar plexus reflex in the centre of the palm.

5 Irritability and mood swings

It is worth just reminding ourselves here, that it is of fundamental importance that a woman listens to and trusts her own inner voice. As discussed earlier, the fluctuations in hormone levels at menopause are similar to the end of the luteal phase of a woman's menstrual cycle, when levels are dropping, and she may experience things that are normally manageable as very irritating. By trusting herself she may use this as a way of finding out how she feels about many aspects of her life.

Besides your whole-body reflexology treatment, areas to give extra attention will be:
- Endocrine system - to balance the hormonal system
- Reproductive system - to help to balance the hormones, so helping mood
- Solar plexus - to help achieve deep relaxation, to lift mood and achieve some clarity of thought
- Diaphragm - to aid deeper breathing to help relaxation and achieve calmness
- Liver 3 *(Figure 5)*
- Gall Bladder 44 *(Figure 9)*

In Chinese Medicine feelings of irritability and frustration are associated with the Wood Element and the meridians associated with this Element are the Liver and Gallbladder. When Wood energy is balanced a person is able to be flexible, creative, and decisive. When it is out of balance they may: feel irritable and frustrated; experience sudden feelings of anger; find it difficult to make decisions; feel apathetic; be self-critical and suffer low self-esteem. Headaches and migraines are also commonly associated with the Wood Element as Liver energy can easily rise up into the head.

Useful tips for helping Wood energy are to:
- Reduce stress
- Express your emotions
- Move your body - any form of exercise especially stretching and particularly the sides of the body where the Liver and Gall Bladder meridians run. Swinging your arms whist twisting from the waist is especially helpful
- Think about your goals for your life and make a plan

Acupressure points

Liver 3

- promotes the smooth flow of Qi around the body *(Figure 5)*
- Gall Bladder 44
- Lateral and proximal to the corner of the 4th toe nail bed. *(Figure 9)*
- Actions:
- Calms the Mind
- Calms Liver Yang

General advice

A bit more about the Kidneys

As I said earlier, the Kidneys are like the batteries of the body. Kidney Yin Deficiency leads to feelings of 'Empty Heat', but the Kidneys are also susceptible to cold and they govern the lower abdominal area (known as the Hara) and the lower back. For this reason, I recommend to most of my clients that they buy a 'Haramaki' or Hara warmer. A Hara warmer is a band of stretchy material which covers you from just above your waist to the top of your hips and keeps your organs and most importantly your Kidneys warm. Most people find that it helps them to feel warmer generally if they feel the cold, and it will help to conserve the Vital Substances stored in the Kidneys. A large scarf can of course also be used.

Yin is nourished by rest and nourishment on physical and psychological levels, so tuning in to our inner selves and developing the ability to go with the flow of our lives is helpful, as is a healthy diet.

Beneficial foods

Fruit and vegetables, pulses, nuts and seeds, wholegrains, seaweeds, seafoods and animal products in small amounts are all helpful to strengthen the Kidneys. Also kidney beans, mung beans, chestnuts, walnuts and parsley are said to 'tonify the Kidneys'.

Foods that are particularly useful for nourishing Kidney Yin are barley, millet and oats, tofu, string beans, asparagus, dark fruits such as blackberries, blueberries, black beans, fish and eggs, dairy produce, sesame seeds, tahini, duck and pork.

Bibliography

Northrupp Christiane, MD (2012) The Wisdom of the Menopause. Bantam Books New York

Beresford-Cooke Carola (2016) Shiatsu Theory and Practice. Third Edition, Singing Dragon

Pitchford Paul (2002) Healing with Wholefoods. Third Edition, North Atlantic Books

Leggett Daverick (2008) Recipes for Self-healing. Meridian Press

Blyth Danny and Lampert Greg (2015) Chinese dietary wisdom, Eating for health and wellbeing. Second edition, Nutshell Press

Horrigan Bonnie. J. (1997) Red Moon Passage, The power and wisdom of Menopause. Thorsons

Thank you for the mentoring on all things Chinese:

Dinah John BA FwSS, Principal of The Shiatsu College Norwich

About Jane Sheehan (Norwich)

At 19 years old, when I first had a massage at a naturopathic clinic, I knew that, some day, I wanted to be involved in complementary therapy - the difference to my sense of wellbeing, physical comfort and mood was remarkable! I trained at St Barts Hospital in London and, after a varied nursing career, I then trained in massage in 1989. I went on to train in a whole range of other bodywork and energy-based practices including Aromatherapy, Reflexology, Reiki, Shiatsu and Qigong.

My burning ambition was to combine my nursing knowledge and my many therapy skills, and I achieved this when I became the first complementary therapy co-ordinator employed at the Specialist Palliative Care Centre in Norwich. I had worked hard to prepare for this by travelling the country to study the provision of therapies for a cancer care setting, without knowing whether such a job would ever become available, so I was over the moon to be working there.

I was awarded the highest accolade of FHT Complementary Therapist of the year 2018 for the work that I did in developing this service, and one of the achievements of which I am most proud is that complementary therapists were subsequently employed by the NHS.

I also practise Hypnotherapy and teach the M Technique and Yoga. One of the most fun things that I do is running Yoga/Qigong holidays abroad, in places such as Greece, Italy and Denmark.

For many years I have had a special interest in working with women's health, from fertility and pregnancy to menopause. I am passionate about helping women to manage these periods in their lives, enabling them to feel relaxed, empowered and able to improve their own health and wellbeing - and I enjoy running a busy clinic doing just that.

I feel so lucky to be able to spend my time doing work that I love. Outside of work I like nothing better than spending time with my family, walking in the countryside with my spaniel Poppy, and I'm often found working at the allotment – or chatting!

Qualifications

Anatomy, Physiology & Massage Diploma 1989

Aromatherapy Diploma 1995

Reflexology Practitioner Certificate 2000

Reiki Level 2 2006

Indian Head Massage Certificate 2006

Professional Hypnotherapy and NLP Diploma (Distinction) 2008

Hypnotherapy for Pregnancy & Childbirth Certificate 2008

Hypnotherapy Practitioner Diploma 2008

Advanced Hypnotherapy & NLP Diploma (Distinction) 2008

Shiatsu Professional Practitioner Diploma 2009

Hypnobirthing Practitioner 2010

M Technique Practitioner 2010

Massage & Cancer Care Practitioner Diploma 2010

Maternity Reflexology Certificate 2010

Clinical Reflexology Post-Grad Diploma in 2011

M Technique Instructor 2013

Qigong Teaching Certificate 2015

Pregnancy Massage Diploma 2015

Fertile Body Therapist 2015

Seren Natural Fertility Reproflexology 2015/2016

Yoga Teacher Training Certificate 2017

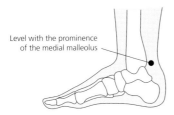

Figure 1: On the medial side of the ankle between the medial malleolus and the Achilles tendon, in the depression level with the tip of the medial malleolus.

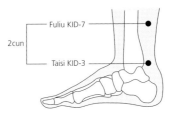

Figure 2: Three fingers proximal to above Kidney 3, on the anterior border of the Achilles tendon.

Figure 3: On the medial side of the foot, 1 thumb's width below the medial malleolus.

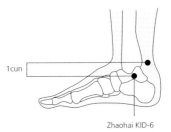

Figure 4: In the depression on the sole of the foot when in plantarflexion, proximal to the junction of the 2nd and 3rd metatarsal heads. (If you slide your thumb just at the lower edge of the reflexology diaphragm reflex you will find a dip in the middle that your thumb will slide into.)

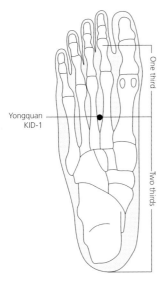

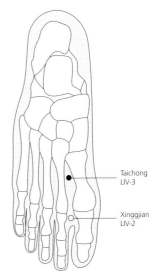

Figure 5: On the dorsum of the foot in the depression just distal to the junction of the first and second metatarsal bones.

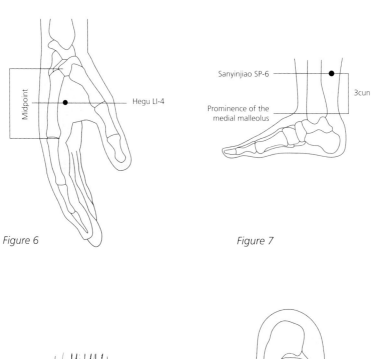

Figure 6

Figure 7

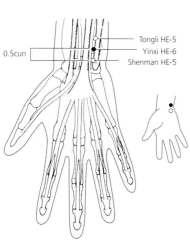

Figure 8

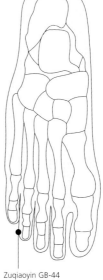

Figure 9

Support for Reflexologists and their Clients

Tips for Successful Breastfeeding
by Maura O'Shea

Top 5 Tips for Successful Breastfeeding
by Maura O'Shea

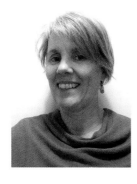

Maura is a Doula, Reflexologist and runs a Breastfeeding Support & Information Group in Tramore, County Waterford (Ireland). Here she shares the top 5 tips for successful breastfeeding as suggested by the mums attending her group:

1. Support Surround yourself with as much breastfeeding support as possible. If things don't seem to be going well at the start, get help as soon as possible from the hospital midwives, hospital/local Lactation Consultant or your local Breastfeeding Counsellor who may be able to visit you in hospital or in the early days at home.

Ask your close family and friends to support you by preparing meals for you, helping with household chores or minding older children over the first few days and weeks so you can concentrate on recovering from pregnancy and labour and getting breastfeeding off to a good start.

2. Information Try to source good research based breastfeeding information from reputable sources such as 'The Womanly Art of Breastfeeding' book, 'The Positive Breastfeeding Book' by Amy Brown or websites such as www.kellymom.com, www.laleche.org.uk, www.nct.org.uk.

3.   Go to a breastfeeding support group while pregnant This has helped many of our local mums as they have found out lots of good information by attending a meet-up before their baby arrives. They also get to meet the local Breastfeeding Counsellor or La Leche League Leader which sometimes makes it easier to contact her to ask for help and information if the need arises! They can also borrow free breastfeeding books from our group library and meet other mums in a lovely, supportive setting.

4. Positioning Recent studies have shown that many babies breastfeed very well in a more Laidback or Natural Breastfeeding position. (Think puppies or piglets lying across their mum!) We too are mammals and in the early days this position seems to stimulate certain reflexes located on the front of a baby's body which in turn encourages baby to open their mouths wide to get a good latch. www.youtu.be/diuGQhbjC6s

5.   Preparation Before baby arrives, batch cook and freeze as many meals as possible to make life as easy as possible in the early weeks! Have some snacks on stand-by such as crackers, rice cakes, yogurts, fruit, hummus, peanut butter, flapjacks, etc.

Some Health Insurance Providers offer free Postpartum Doula hours to help mums in the early days and weeks so check out your insurance just in case!

To find your local Breastfeeding Support Group:
www.laleche.org.uk/find-lll-support-group/
www.nct.org.uk/local-activities-meet-ups/local-parent-support
www.lalecheleagueireland.com/groups/
https://www.cuidiu.ie/supports_breastfeeding

Hope that helps and best wishes to you and your little one!

About Maura O'Shea

Maura O'Shea is a Breastfeeding Counsellor and has run a support group on a voluntary basis for over 13 years in Waterford (Ireland). During this time, she has assisted many mothers on their breastfeeding journey by providing research based breastfeeding information, help and support through monthly meet-ups whilst also operating a helpline.

For the past couple of years, she has also been working as a Postpartum Doula where she supports mums in those precious but exhausting early days and weeks of motherhood. Maura feels that 'mothering the mother' during this period is so important to assist recovery from pregnancy and birth both physically and mentally.

Maura is also a qualified Reflexologist with a special interest in fertility, pregnancy and women's health.

She lives by the sea in Tramore, Co. Waterford with her husband and two teenage children.

To find out more please contact Maura at:
tramorereflexology@gmail.com
www.facebook.com/tramorereflexology/

Lifestyle Choices for A Healthy Mind and Body During Menopause

by Teri Woods

Lifestyle Choices for A Healthy Mind and Body During Menopause
by Teri Woods

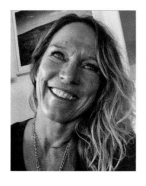

The age a woman experiences menopause varies, it typically occurs during her late forties or early fifties. However, symptoms of menopause may begin well before menstruation stops (perimenopause). Genetics, individual biochemistry and lifestyle all play a role in the age menopause starts[1]. No matter what age a woman is at the onset, she can experience a myriad of symptoms that significantly affect her physical and mental wellbeing.

In perimenopausal or menopausal women, the symptoms may include:

- Hot flashes
- Vaginal dryness
- Interstitial cystitis
- Painful intercourse
- Insomnia
- Low libido
- Anxiety
- Mood swings
- Depression
- Irritability
- Decrease in bone density
- Dry, itchy skin
- Inflammation/joint pain
- Brain fog
- Hair loss
- IBS (Irritable Bowel Syndrome)

Most often when women talk about perimenopause or menopause it is about the rollercoaster of symptoms they are experiencing, which can be tiresome, frustrating and anxiety producing. Whilst it's not always possible for women to avoid symptoms of menopause entirely, there are ways to ease the transition. The severity of symptoms depends on various contributing factors including, smoking, alcohol, obesity, sedentary lifestyle, poor diet, stress and exposure to toxins.

Every woman is unique, so it goes without saying their experience of menopause will be unique as well. Women have access to more grace, wisdom and power during this time in life. However, when overcome with symptoms that are wreaking havoc on their bodies and minds it is challenging to appreciate the liberating aspects of the process.

Practitioners have the potential to create great value for women during these years. Empowering them with information, encouraging them to be open-minded and curious, enables them to take responsibility for their own health and wellbeing. Natural and holistic approaches along with diet and lifestyle changes are highly effective in reducing the severity and impact of the symptoms related to menopause. Here are a few that are well researched and always show up at the top of the list.

Eat Nutrient Dense Foods – Limit Trigger Foods

Dietary imbalances and poor lifestyle choices can lead to women experiencing more severe symptoms during menopause. Encouraging them to adopt healthier habits prior to the onset of menopause can make a significant difference in mitigating these symptoms.

When fatigue, insomnia, and moodiness are present it can lead to skipping meals and poor food choices as well as excessive sugar, caffeine, and alcohol intake. All these substances are known triggers that may exacerbate hormone fluctuations, hot flashes, mood swings, and depression. Eating regular meals full of unprocessed whole foods including organic vegetables, grains and quality protein help stabilize blood sugar levels which can limit cravings. This approach can assist women with less weight gain, reduced fatigue and more balanced moods.

Most practitioners working with women during this transition advise eliminating processed foods. Prepacked and prepared foods are typically full of high levels of unhealthy fat, excess sodium and sugar. These foods can contribute to inflammation, high cholesterol, elevated blood pressure and diabetes to name a few. Encourage women to schedule extra time to cook healthy meals at home. Also, cooking and freezing extra portions for the days they are lacking energy and not motivated to cook is a great way to ensure healthy meals are always available.

As well as eating regular meals, healthy snacks in between meals can be helpful in reducing mood swings. Serotonin is sometimes at the root of these mood swings since it is the neurotransmitter that helps regulate mood, body temperature, and appetite. When levels run low, women are more likely to be irritable and crave sugar, a quick snack can be a great mood elevator. Snack choices should be well-balanced with good levels of complex carbohydrates, protein and healthy fat.

As ovaries produce less and less oestrogen, the bones begin to thin faster and the risk of osteoporosis and fractures increases.[2] Incorporating dairy products as a regular part of the diet is recommended. Advise sources such as low-fat milk, cheese, and yogurt; always local and organic when possible. For women who are allergic or have a dairy intolerance, advise adding more foods that are naturally high in calcium. Many leafy greens can increase calcium intake including broccoli, spinach, kale, bok choy, turnip greens and collard greens. Also, dried figs, chia seeds and sesame seeds are other excellent non-dairy sources of calcium.

During this time and as a woman becomes postmenopausal, it is often necessary to include a supplement with calcium, in conjunction with Vitamin D3 and K2. These nutrients assist with maintaining healthy calcium levels and optimizing bone metabolism which reduces the risk of osteoporosis. This is a vital component for women to be aware of during this transition, and best for them to seek guidance from a practitioner working in this field.

Including foods rich in omega-3s in the diet is always beneficial and specifically for these years of a woman's life. This essential fatty acid improves cardiovascular function, brain health and helps with a healthy oil barrier in the skin which improves the symptoms related to dry skin.[3] Besides seafood, other whole food sources with high levels of omega-3 are walnuts, chia seeds, hemp seeds and ground flaxseed or flax meal. (Remember, it's best to choose wild seafood over farmed when possible.)

Keep in mind that the dietary and nutritional needs may be quite different from woman to woman.

Encouraging intuitive eating to learn what feels nourishing and appropriate for their bodies can empower women and help them take responsibility for their health and wellbeing. In cases where digestive distress is an issue suggest relaxed eating (no rushing), sitting down during meals, chewing food well and keeping a food journal. These steps will increase self-awareness during meals and help determine what food intolerances or sensitivities may be present.

There are many websites containing whole food recipes for snacks, meals and desserts. Creating a list of these sites can be a valuable resource for your clients to assist them with being creative in the kitchen and making healthy food choices.

Hydration

The human body is composed of over 65% water. Every day water plays a major role maintaining and supporting healthy cells and body's vital organs. During menopause decreased levels of oestrogen contribute to dryness throughout the body, therefore proper hydration becomes even more crucial during perimenopause and menopause.[4] Common symptoms related to dehydration include hot flashes, brain fog, constipation, dry skin and joint pain. The average recommendation for adult water intake is 64 ounces a day (1.8L). However, current research advises individuals drink half of their bodyweight in ounces per day. A few other factors that can increase the need for additional hydration during menopause may include women suffering from hot flashes and night sweats, avid exercisers and those living in warm climates. Also, how quickly water is consumed makes a big difference in how effectively the body is hydrated. Sipping water throughout the day versus gulping down 16 ounces (454ml) or more at a time has been shown to lead to more optimal hydration and less stress on the kidneys.[5]

Infusing water with fresh fruit and herbs is a great way to increase water intake. Also, adding fruits and vegetables to the diet that have high water contents will boost daily hydration. A few recommendations are: lettuce, spinach, kale, tomatoes, cucumbers, celery, zucchini (courgetti), broccoli, cauliflower, radishes, melons, berries and pineapple.

Practise gratitude & mindfulness

During menopause, lower amounts of oestrogen and progesterone leave women less able to cope with stress. The effect of stress alone can be so intense that it can induce and increase the severity of symptoms. Lack of concentration, irrational thinking, digestive issues, weight gain and sleep problems are all common side effects. The cascading effect of stress on the brain and body in conjunction with the symptoms of menopause is a setup for the onset of chronic illness. Therefore, finding effective techniques to manage stress is an essential part of a menopause protocol.

Maintaining a positive outlook when all the negative impacts of perimenopause or menopause are raging can be challenging. Research is producing strong evidence that some simple, yet effective techniques can ease the stress, anxiety and discomfort associated with some of the more common mental and physical symptoms. Self-care plays an essential role in managing stress during menopause. Spending time alone, cultivating gratitude and practising mindfulness through journaling, yoga or meditation are all excellent choices. When women take even 15 minutes a day to make themselves a priority, dramatic changes can occur. This approach to wellbeing must be done with consistency for maximum benefits, addressing emotional, physical, and spiritual needs. When women take the time to make themselves a priority, nagging symptoms decrease and the possibility of a positive experience during this transition increases.

Starting a gratitude journal can be a valuable part of a self-care routine. Practising gratitude on a regular basis increases positive emotions while reducing anxiety and depression.[6] The act of consciously composing and directing thoughts helps brings thoughts to the present moment. Acknowledging and appreciating simple everyday things can help limit the impact of stress.

Certain types of yoga, specifically restorative and gentle hatha, relieve stress and alleviate other common symptoms of menopause.[7] Through breath and movement, yoga helps balance the nervous system, which increases the coordination between the body and the mind. A key component of yoga is pranayama, or the Sanskrit word for "controlled breathing." Pranayama helps quiet the mind and create a calmer mental state overall. Maintaining a daily yoga practice, even a few times a week, can lead to a more positive outlook, mental clarity and improved sleep. To avoid injury, it is best to be introduced to yoga through a class in a studio setting as opposed to using an online resource. Women with knee, hip, or shoulder problems should consult with a certified yoga instructor prior to attempting any poses.

Meditation is another great option for self-care routines to reduce stress and anxiety. Taking the brain off autopilot and sitting quietly without judgement, letting thoughts come and go, is a practice that improves over time. The parasympathetic nervous system is activated during meditation which means the whole body shifts into a calming state. This ability to calm the mind enables women to be more resilient towards stress and disassociate from their symptoms, and over time connect to inner strength. Numerous studies validate the positive benefits of meditation, including better overall brain function, healthier cardiovascular function, reduced systemic inflammation, improved sleep and better immune function.[8] For the many attributes of a daily practice to be realized, it only requires a minimal commitment of 15 minutes. A guided practice is best if someone is new to meditation.

Stay Active

Weight gain during menopause is common and can have serious implications on women's health including increased risk of heart disease and type 2 diabetes. Extra weight has also been shown to exacerbate both physical and psychological symptoms. It is well documented that exercise improves heart and brain function, increases metabolism, reduces stress, releases endorphins that boost mood and improves sleep.[9] All of these areas are impacted during menopause, which is why regular exercise can be very beneficial in reducing some of the most common, bothersome symptoms. Even if a woman is currently sedentary, overweight, and dealing with rough symptoms, starting to exercise now is a smart move. In one study, women in both perimenopause and post menopause who had sedentary lifestyles began exercising moderately three days a week for 12 weeks. All participants reported improved sleep quality and mood compared to a control group.

One of the most common symptoms are hot flashes, approximately 75% of menopausal women experience them. Believe it or not, breaking a sweat regularly and increasing the intensity of exercise over time, helps blood vessels become more efficient at carrying heat to the surface of skin and releasing it. One study clearly illustrates how effective exercise can be in mitigating this symptom. Researchers asked women experiencing hot flashes to participate in a 16-week exercise program. The program gradually increased the intensity of workouts until participants were jogging or biking at a sweat-inducing clip for 45 minutes, four or five times a week. At the four- month mark women reported at least a 60% reduction in hot flashes[10].

Another important type of exercise for women to strongly consider adding to their lives during this time is strength training. Weight-bearing exercises such as weight lifting and activities done standing up like walking, running, jogging, dancing, aerobics, and racquet sports are excellent ways to increase bone mass and build bone density.[11] Therefore, including resistance training a couple times a week is an excellent preventative for osteoporosis. When a woman is new to exercise, encourage her to seek the advice of a professional to find out what type of exercise will be most beneficial for her body.

Adaptogenic herbs help the body adapt

Due to the impact of fluctuating hormones, stress can be prevalent during all stages of menopause, creating a cascade of irritating physical and mental effects throughout the body. When chronic stress is ignored it weakens the immune system which can be an opening for illness to occur. Adaptogenic herbs have the unique ability to "adapt" to the body's needs, restoring balance and building a healthier response to stress.[12] These restorative properties play a key role in reducing the physical and mental stress of perimenopause and menopause. Including them in a protocol in conjunction with a healthy diet and lifestyle adds much needed foundational support towards sustaining a healthy body and mind. Examples of researched adaptogens that are safe and proven to be very effective in reducing the most common symptoms are: holy basil, ashwaghanda, schisandra, rhodiola and maca.

Herbal supplements are not closely regulated in all countries; it is important to note that the quality, safety, and purity may vary between brands. As with all therapies, there are potential risks and/ or side effects. Also, herbal therapies may interact with prescription drugs, resulting in dramatic changes in the effect of the botanical, the drug, or both. To be safe, always consult with a licensed practitioner prior to beginning a protocol.

Address imbalances

In order for many of the common dietary and holistic approaches towards menopause to be truly effective, underlying health issues need to be addressed first. For example, when the diet lacks basic nutrients and gut issues are present, the ratio of good versus bad bacteria is out of balance which can reduce circulating oestrogen. Micronutrient deficiencies, adrenal insufficiency, or thyroid issues may also be present and need to be treated to reestablish better overall health. It is always advisable for a woman to have a practitioner/ naturopath experienced in functional medicine and women's health to assist them through this journey.

Honour the process

Menopause is a powerful transformation; a time for women to get curious about what enlivens and empowers them. The attitude a woman has towards the changes occurring in her body will create the biggest difference in her experience. A woman spends a lot of her life nurturing and caring for others. Menopause is a time to reprioritize and redirect that love, and really start nurturing herself. A time to trust instincts, rebuild the confidence in her mind and body. A beautiful and deep understanding unfolds, allowing her innate wisdom to guide her through life with grace and ease.

About Teri Woods

Teri Woods, CCN, CHC at IN2U Healthy Living (in2urhealth.com)

Teri is a clinical nutritionist and health coach who loves working in partnership with women; empowering and enlivening them to live healthy, fulfilling lives. Working in the field of health and well-being for over 25 years, she is a firm believer that there is no "one size fits all" approach to optimal health. She follows her natural curiosity to determine what type of nourishment each woman's body and mind need to thrive and come alive.

Contact Teri via her website **www.trubodymind.com**

References:

1 https://www.ncbi.nlm.nih.gov/pmc/articles/PMC3955043/

2 https://pubmed.ncbi.nlm.nih.gov/21179049/

3 https://www.sciencedaily.com/releases/2009/01/090128104702.htm

4 https://www.ncbi.nlm.nih.gov/pmc/articles/PMC2908954/

5 https://www.sciencedirect.com/science/article/pii/S008525381550495X

6 https://www.ncbi.nlm.nih.gov/pmc/articles/PMC3010965/

7 https://www.ncbi.nlm.nih.gov/pmc/articles/PMC3122509/

8 https://www.ncbi.nlm.nih.gov/pmc/articles/PMC3031101/

9 https://www.ncbi.nlm.nih.gov/pmc/articles/PMC4828504/

10 https://pubmed.ncbi.nlm.nih.gov/27163520/

11 https://pubmed.ncbi.nlm.nih.gov/28017948/

12 https://www.ncbi.nlm.nih.gov/pmc/articles/PMC6240259/

Aromatherapy and Reflexology for the Menopause

by Beverley Higham

Aromatherapy and Reflexology for the Menopause
by Beverley Higham

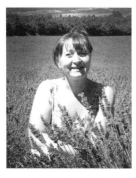

As I write this it is *Lavender Season* in Provence. July is a highly aromatic season when the air is full of the sweet lavender fragrance as the plants are distilled to release the soothing, stress relieving essence of the pure essential oil. Distillation is the process of releasing the healing oil from the plant. Bundles of cut and sun-dried flowers are packed tightly into the still. Steam is then introduced which rises through the plant material and, as it ascends it takes the volatile aromatic molecules with it. The steam reaches the condenser where it cools and is returned to its liquid state. The now flower-scented water collects in a beaker, causing the light fragrant lavender essential oil to float to the surface. The essential oil will be drained off and stored in a cool dark place, ready to be bottled. The flower water will become lavender hydrolat which will be used in toiletries and cosmetics. Visiting Provence in the summer months allows visitors to witness this process and join in the various flower festivals. The town of Grasse, an hour from Nice, was once the perfume capital of the world. It is the gateway to a fairy land of fragrance and *aromatherapy*, and this is where I have learnt my art!

The word aroma means 'smell' or 'fragrance' and *therapy* means 'treatment' – so *aromatherapy* is a 'fragrant treatment'. Our nose plays a vital role in the process and this is where the greatest impact can be made. As we inhale pleasing fragrant aromas, the cilia in our olfactory bulb at the back of the nose pick up the tiny molecules and, like keys turning in locks, the pathway to the neuro transmitters in the brain are opened and "pow!" we have the real effect of aromatherapy just as it was intended possibly by the flower itself? Suddenly our body feels the soothing effects as our own natural endorphins and encephalin are released: our limbic system, said to be the seat of all emotion, transports us to lavender fields from long forgotten memories, or puts us in the rose-scented arms of our grandmothers and we are children once more. Essential oils can stimulate the oldest part of our brain: this is where the real treatment starts. Aromatherapy is a body, mind and spirit treatment; that is what makes it truly holistic. By spirit we mean the charisma, personality and essential part of what makes a person who they are and how they interact with life. We often refer to the term "high spirited", or "low in spirit". Aromatherapy can revive the spirit, because just like the petals of the flowers we obtain essential oils from, we humans open and close depending on our moods and emotions. We have such synergy with essential oils because we are part of the same whole, life itself!

That is why fragrance is so satisfying to human beings. We are led by our noses in more ways than you may realise. Our noses recognise people by smells. The aroma of food can stimulate our digestive system and a sultry aroma can bring romance to the air.

I use aromatherapy in all my treatments and below I will discuss the use of aromatherapy for some of the conditions that may be of interest to you in your therapy work.

Aromatherapy and reflexology for the menopause

The menopause marks the end of the physical reproductive phase of a woman's life: in most cases it begins around the age of 45 and ends by 55 years of age, although this can vary.

During this time women may experience many changes such as:

- Body fat from the hips and thighs redistributed to the stomach and back
- Hair, nails and skin become dry without the softening effects of oestrogen
- Night sweats and hot flushes which last for weeks, months or even longer
- Feeling more emotional, weepy and having a poor self- image. This can even be accompanied by 'brain fog', forgetfulness and memory issues

Aromatherapy can be beneficial for these distressing and unpleasant symptoms. It can be used in harmony with reflexology during treatment but also offered to the client as part of their self-help routine. Below is a list of the oils I have found most useful:

Vetiver (vetiveria zizanoides)

In my experience this oil - known in India as the 'oil of tranquillity' - can be highly beneficial when night sweats are disrupting normal sleep patterns. Cooling and grounding, it can act as a sedative to the nervous system. It blends well with clary sage and sandalwood and aids restful sleep. Sleep can be disturbed due to hot flushes and night sweats. In India vetiver is used to make blinds in buildings and fans to waft away the heat. It is highly effective for its cooling properties. The oil is also said to be ideal for masculine ageing. It is always nice when I can mention this as aromatherapy is often seen as a predominantly female treatment.

Vetiver can be blended into an unscented lotion base at a 1% blend which is approx. 20 drops of essential oil to 100 ml of base lotion. This is ideal to use during reflexology treatment or the client can massage their own feet before bed. This is a very self-nurturing thing to do and helps to ground the energy and aid sleep. It is a very calming oil and I have used it with clients during consultation when clients have a lot of nervous energy causing them to be overly talkative when really, they need silence and relaxation.

Petitgrain (citrus aurantium)

This is useful for emotional transitions caused by the menopause. Blended with frankincense it can help alleviate anxiety and nervous exhaustion, it deepens the breath. It is also useful for excessive perspiration. It can be vaporised in the treatment room or recommended to the client to use at home. The essential oils (5 drops of each if using both oils) can be diluted in a little alcohol (approx. 1 tsp) and added to water to make a room spray. Shake the bottle before spraying into the room. It can also be used in the car before travelling, aiding a calm environment for safe travel.

Rose (rosa damascena)

My clients have found this truly luxurious aroma helpful in restoring libido and re-building self-confidence. It can be used to help improve the condition of mature sensitive skins. Rose is said to be the closest fragrance to the natural scent of a woman. During the menopause this exotic flower can help to strengthen the feminine confidence which often appears to be fading at this time. It is a highly expensive oil but one well worth the investment. Rose hydrolat is another valuable cosmetic at this time of life. It makes a fabulous skin tonic, helping to reduce redness of the facial skin which often accompanies the menopause. I even use rose water in my steam iron so that as I press the clothes, I receive a little aromatherapy at the same time. The clothes smell wonderful too.

Clary Sage (salvia sclarea)

This is a deeply relaxing and stress-relieving oil. It can help to ease anxiety and nervous tension whilst uplifting the spirit. It can aid sleep when blended with lavender: a couple of drops on the pillow or dilute it in base oil and massage it into your client's feet after reflexology to aid a restful night's sleep. As with all essential oils and treatments it is best to ensure that no alcohol is consumed after aromatherapy and especially when using clary sage. It is a powerful oil and could cause nightmares if alcohol is consumed when using this oil.

It blends well with lavender, geranium, bergamot and other citrus oils. It's a great oil to use for the changes at this period in a woman's life as it is said to mimic oestrogen in its chemical makeup.

Aromatic waters

Aromatic waters such as the previously mentioned rose water, are also effective in helping menopausal conditions. They are uplifting, cooling, refreshing and can be carried in a spritzer spray to combat hot flushes or power surges during the day.

Bitter orange flower water has a sedative action and is traditionally used for anxiety. It can also be used as a skin tonic - it has moisturising and rejuvenating properties. It can help to improve the dry skin that many menopausal women may experience. During a reflexology session you can use these, following feet sanitising, or at the end of a treatment to refresh the feet, leaving the client and the room pleasantly fragrant.

Case studies

Below is a summary of two treatments I conducted for menopausal clients whilst working within my local practice. The clients were referred to me by their GP. There were specific reasons why their doctor wanted to try a more complementary approach.

Woman aged 54 years

Symptoms - tension headaches, stress, difficulty sleeping, hot flushes, arthritic knee, constipation and varicose veins.

Current medication - HRT patches (Doctor's permission received).

Selected oils – a base of lime blossom macerate (antispasmodic/sedative). The lime blossoms are soaked in a vegetable-based oil and over the course of a few weeks the oil absorbs the therapeutic properties of the blossoms; it is a beautiful base oil for pain. I combined the oil with a base lotion. To this was added vetiver, ylang ylang, benzoin and clary sage. The oils were to be applied nightly to the upper body and during the day to the abdomen and legs.

Result – the client had better sleep, fewer tension headaches, and her stress and anxiety were reduced. Circulation improved due to application of lotion to the legs. Overall, the client felt refreshed and more balanced. Part of the success of any treatment such as this is the empowerment of the client. Making them part of the treatment and its application is especially important to the overall success. Visiting a reflexologist or aromatherapist is an excellent experience and a good investment in personal wellbeing, but it's what you do between visits that is just as important to overall health.

Woman aged 60 years (still experiencing menopausal-like symptoms)

Symptoms - hot flushes, night sweats also occurring during the morning, anxiety and depression.

Current medication - none, GP referred her immediately for aromatherapy and reflexology treatment.

Selected oils - bergamot, geranium and rose. These were blended in a white base lotion to be applied to the upper body after a morning shower. A second blend of frankincense, sandalwood and ylang ylang with base oil was provided for the client to apply before bed.

Result - the daytime anxiety and day sweats quickly diminished but she still experienced the night sweats. I, therefore, changed the evening blend to petitgrain, neroli and rose, blended in white base lotion and sweet almond oil. This brought a reduction to the frequency of night sweats. Night sweats are a challenge; I suffered terribly but thanks to aromatherapy there is often help at hand, but they can lead to sleep loss and fatigue. Perseverance will lead to a decline. Every client is different and therefore what suits one does not always suit another, although you will often see a commonality in the choices of oils from clients suffering with similar symptoms.

Combining aromatherapy with reflexology

The medical profession is beginning to realise how effective aromatherapy and reflexology can be, especially where modern medicine has been unable to help. By empowering our clients with the pleasant use of aromatherapy blends and natural ingredients we can bring greater balance and significantly improve their health and wellbeing. Reflexology is a wonderful tool for introducing the use of essential oils and encouraging the client to continue with home care procedures to manage their day to day life changes.

Time to pause – this was the name I gave to a blend I created for treating my clients who were reaching the menopause. It was a blend of four essential oils. I chose each of them to represent the experiences of a woman approaching menopause. I have had great success with the blend but also add to it when I feel a client requires additional oils.

Jasmine (jasminum officinale) – A very heavy, sweet and exotic floral scent. The significance of this oil is that it blooms at twilight. Its heavenly fragrance is apparent as dusk approaches and I felt that this oil represents the woman approaching menopause. We too can bloom in our twilight years: menopause does not need to be the end of our femininity! We can bloom like jasmine. The oil is an aphrodisiac. It is what many of us need at this time as loss of libido can be experienced during menopause.

Mandarin (citrus reticulata) - this oil helps us to find our joy! Often as we reach this part of our lives, our children have flown the nest, and we have settled into our careers so now it is time for us to find ourself and what brings us joy? Mandarin oil can help us to do this. It has an uplifting and energising fragrance.

Vetiver (vetiver zizanoides) - as already discussed earlier in the chapter, this oil is grounding and cooling. It also has a message for us. As our skin starts to lose elasticity as the collagen and elastin fibres slacken in age, this oil is said to help give our skin its bounce back. The actual grass itself is grown in subtropical regions to prevent land slide after the rains. So, let's give it a go and see if it can help keep our skin from sliding too!

Lime (citrus aurantifolia) – I chose this oil as, not only does it have a zesty fragrance like lemon, but it is said to cleanse negativity from our aura. Often, we hold on to negative feelings or begin to feel negative as if our femininity is fading with the menopause. This oil will pick us up, dust us off and reset us on our way. Many of my clients have found benefit from this blend. I use it around the home. It can be diluted in base oil for massage and one of my clients uses it on the reproductive reflexes on her feet and all around the ankles. This, she tells, me keeps her flushes at bay.

Men and aromatherapy

Men benefit from aromatherapy too. We have already mentioned how rose oil helps confidence, but it is also said to help with sperm! It is an aphrodisiac so let's not cast off that possibility. Men who are terribly busy and have lives that are stressful benefit from a regular professional aromatherapy massage or reflexology to balance and harmonise the body and mind. The use of aromatherapy eases the symptoms of stress: it helps release tension and improve the circulation.

- Woody aromas like cedarwood and sandalwood are highly appealing to men and often used in male fragrance. They ease emotional stress and have a grounding effect.
- Fruity fragrances like lemon and grapefruit are uplifting and energising. These oils help to restore motivation.
- Herbaceous aromas like basil and rosemary are stress relieving and ease muscle tension.
- Exotic heavy aromas aid sleep and are relaxing. Never underestimate the power of the flower for men as well as women.

A blend of black pepper, ylang ylang and ginger can re-light the inner fire and bring passion back where loss of libido adds pressure to a relationship. It is not only menopausal women who may need help with libido. Adding 2 drops of each oil to 20 ml of sweet almond or sunflower oil and massaging the lower back and legs works like magic! But it is advisable to let the client use this blend with their partner. Black pepper is a stimulating, warming oil. It is contraindicated for clients with high blood pressure. Ylang ylang is a floral note. It reduces anxiety and is calming and aphrodisiac. Ginger is warming, it improves the circulation. It relaxes the muscles. The blend is generally an excellent massage blend but where a boost is needed in the bedroom this can help. It must, however, not be massaged anywhere near the genitals. Stick to the lower back and thighs only.

One of my male clients suffers from rheumatoid arthritis and finds essential oils wonderful for pain relief. Eucalyptus, peppermint and juniper berry in sunflower oil ease his pain and swelling. He uses this blend on his hands and I use it for reflexology on his feet. He is an advocate of aromatherapy and would never go anywhere without tea tree oil. He preaches its value. He loves to go fishing when he feels well enough as it's like meditation to him. If he gets bothered by flies, or even bitten by a flying insect a dab of tea tree oil rectifies the itchy spot.

Aromatherapy really is for everyone. Men benefit greatly on so many levels and men - just like women - need some therapeutic care, too.

Always seek out the advice of a professional aromatherapist if this is not your specialism or contact me on the links provided. There are many essential oils as we live in a highly aromatic world. There are more exciting oils being discovered and new treatments emerging to aid us in extending our treatment portfolio.

I believe that the best way with aromatherapy is to follow your nose as it really is like an inner compass.

About Beverley Higham

Beverley is a brilliant therapist with over thirty years' experience, and she is humble with it – as many of us therapists are. In fact, she took some persuading to write this chapter: 'I'm not a guru'. But there is not much that Beverley does not know when it comes to aromatherapy, and she has a network of other highly skilled colleagues from her work, study, teaching and play with aromatherapy - and other therapies as well - to direct you to if you need further guidance.

She is a reflexologist and incorporates aromatherapy into her treatments. But it is her therapeutic use of aromatherapy – or as she likes to say, 'The Power of the Flower!' – which is Beverley's passion and 'guru' expertise.

So, what's this humble therapist's background? She initially trained in aromatherapy in 1988 and reflexology was included as part of her training. She completed further training with Sandra Day in the 1990s. Since then, she has completed aromatherapy for cancer training at the Royal Marsden with Rhiannon Lewis, as well as further clinical aromatherapy study in France, also with Rhiannon. She has a BA in Education and is a member of IFPA.

Her experience with cancer care started in 1989 when she did some initial teaching at Wigan Hospice for the staff and Marie Curie nurses; they then went on to complete further training with her at Wigan and Leigh College. She nursed her father through two episodes of cancer and has friends who she has supported through their breast cancer journeys. In the early 1990s she worked with NHS doctors to introduce aromatherapy alongside conventional medicine in her local community.

This led to her publishing some of her research on women's health in the International Journal of Clinical Aromatherapy (Higham, 2008). She has published a guide to aromatherapy including topics on aromatherapy for pregnancy, babies and young children, the menopause, oral hygiene, beauty secrets, and love (Higham, 2015).

Beverley has recently retired after 30 years as a course manager at Wigan and Leigh College, where she ran a Foundation Degree in Spa Management. During her time there she was awarded a Medal of Excellence from City and Guilds.

She was co-founder and creative director of a range of natural organic face, body and spa products. She now creates bespoke products for private and professional clients. She teaches at home in the UK and each summer in Provence, where she runs a retreat in the heart of the lavender growing region.

She is currently writing her second book on the art of creating natural plant-based cosmetics.

If you would like to get in contact with Beverley, please email her on:
b.higham@hotmail.co.uk or
Info@beverleyhigham.co.uk
guidehttp://beverleyhigham.co.uk/
https://beverleyhigham.co.uk

Further reading

HIGHAM, B., 2008. Essential Oil Interventions for Premenstrual Syndrome and the Menopause: Experiences of a British aromatherapist. *International Journal of Clinical Aromatherapy*. 5 (2), pp. 35–41.

HIGHAM, B., 2015. *Inspirational Aromatherapy: The Writings of Beverley Higham*. Bloomington, IN: Balboa Press.

Disclaimer

This chapter does not aim to dispense medical advice or prescribe any alternative to orthodox medicine. My intent is only to offer information of a general nature and from my own experience working within my professional boundaries. In the event you use any of the information please do so following the advice of a qualified aromatherapist or your physician. Both myself and the publisher assume no responsibility for your actions. We solely aim to provide inspiration.

Traditional Acupuncture and How it Benefits Fertility

by Amanda Thomas

Traditional Acupuncture and How it Benefits Fertility
by Amanda Thomas

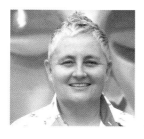

The HEART is profoundly important in Chinese Medicine, as it plays a role in the formation of menstrual blood and, via the internal pathways of the meridians (which are channels of energy), is connected to the Uterus. It's a beautiful reminder that all things are ultimately connected. The body is like a matrix. We all inherit our particular gene set (blueprint) from our parents. However, when we are born, we are also given the gift of 'free will' which enables us to move through life, making choices. The quality of our choices will determine the state of our health and this also affects our fertility. We know this and there is always the opportunity to improve our choices and our fertility levels. At times, depending on our conditioning and the people around us to influence our choices, we may make unhealthy choices or get stuck in ways of being that don't necessarily serve us. We may worry too much, or try to 'people please', get too angry, feel frustrated or resentment towards others. We may feel sorry for or insecure about ourselves and what we think we can achieve. What I have learned as I have moved through my own life and what I have seen through my many years of practice is …. we (already) are what we seek. Acupuncture allows our system to come back into balance and this will affect the way we feel and the decisions we make.

- We can inadvertently give our power away.
- We can override our own wisdom.
- When we 'wake up' to the truth of who we are and the power we have as women, this alone can change the world.

So if you are struggling to conceive. Trust me I know how that feels, having conceived my first child as if by magic but then struggling to conceive and miscarrying during the next 6 years. The important thing is to get support, don't be on your own with everything. Find a practitioner that you feel comfortable with, who you feel heard by, and who will support you on your journey.

The HEART governs Blood - so basically, if there are any emotional factors, such as anxiety, insecurity, feelings of low self-worth, worry, guilt and general over thinking, this will affect the flow of Qi (energy) and affect the flow of Blood too. We may not be conscious of how we are feeling, but the Heart always knows, and this will impact on the state of your health and fertility levels.

When we are weighed down in our experience we can not always see a way out. The light at the end of the tunnel appears very far away. Our hopes and dreams of realising a child can feel a million miles away. Remember the journey of 10,000 miles always starts with one step. Unbeknownst to us, it only takes one thought or a moment to transform our experience of the world and our so-called problems. When you feel ready to take that step, reach out to a practitioner who will guide you on your journey.

What we are looking for is a state of no thought. In our Western way, we can strive towards our goals thinking we need to DO or BE more. We actually need to learn to take our foot off the gas. In this way, LESS is MORE. The vastness of what is available to us is beyond our intellect.

When we are weighed down in our experience we can not always see a way out. The light at the end of the tunnel appears very far away. Our hopes and dreams of realising a child can feel a million miles away. Remember the journey of 10,000 miles always starts with one step. Unbeknownst to us, it only takes one thought or a moment to transform our experience of the world and our so-called problems. When you feel ready to take that step, reach out to a practitioner who will guide you on your journey.

What we are looking for is a state of no thought. An empty mind where peace and the answer to all everything lays. In our Western way, we can strive towards our goals thinking we need to DO or BE more. We actually need to learn to take our foot off the gas. In this way, LESS is MORE. The vastness of what is available to us is beyond our intellect.

So as a practitioner, I provide the space where you can be quiet and it allows you to become more in tune with your own intuition. The answers you need are already inside you. It is just my job to point you in the right direction, which is always inwards. By accepting where you are, without judgement, in a space of neutrality, a space where you feel held metaphorically, there is the opportunity to transform everything.

Out of NOTHING (the spaciousness); comes EVERYTHING (all the answers you need).

So the acupuncture treatment provides the opportunity to relax around everything; to stop making yourself wrong for wherever you are and a welcome pause. Within that pause there is space - within that space is the infinite intelligence behind life.

In a world of over complication, it is important to keep things as simple as you can:

- Focus on what you want
- Find a practitioner that you resonate with who can support the process with you
- Trust - then let go of control; hand it over

Unexplained infertility

If you have been given a diagnosis of 'unexplained infertility,' do not give up hope of conceiving naturally. Chinese Medicine looks at the whole system differently to Western Medicine. There may be factors that can't be explained in a Western sense. A combination of acupuncture and herbal medicine may address issues that have not been identified even after extensive tests. You have everything to gain by at least trying a course of acupuncture treatment. Even if you are afraid of needles, your practitioner can apply acupressure to the points and over time you may build up confidence in your practitioner to try the needles. Most people associate the needles with syringe type needles. They are much finer than that and every patient I have worked with is surprised at how it doesn't hurt in the way they anticipate. I also treat babies and children with a gentle Japanese style of acupuncture called Shonishin. These techniques can also be used on a nervous adult! Gaining confidence and trust in your practitioner is paramount to the success of your treatment. This all happens over the first few treatments. Trust is the key factor. When we trust and are open to the Universe - magic happens! Life is a mystery and I have seen this reflected in my practice. What we know only accounts for 4% - the other 96% is a mystery. I see it as my role to get you, as the patient, to embrace the unknown.

Acupuncture points to support fertility

There are over 200 acupuncture points. Here is a selection of points that will support fertility and prepare the body towards pregnancy.

Lu-7 Lieque (Broken Sequence) + Kid 6 Zhaohai (Shining Sea)

This combination of points regulates the conception vessel (the Ren Mai) which is essential to support pregnancy.

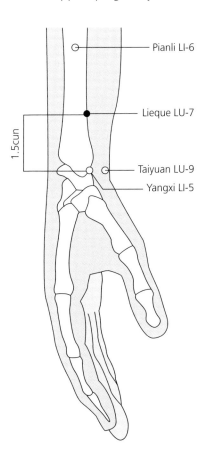

Sp-6 Sanyinjiao (Three Yin Intersection)

This point is a meeting point for all the yin channels (Spleen, Liver and Kidney). It is one of the most important and widely used points. It harmonises and tonifies the Blood. It is very important to tonify this point if there are any disorders of the Blood in the menstrual cycle. These may be indicated by clots on the blood during the period and if there is any period pain which is stagnation of the Qi and the Blood.

Sp-6 is only used to prepare the woman's body for pregnancy or regulate any menstrual irregularities. It is not needled during the pregnancy as it has a strong effect and can cause miscarriage. It can be used at the end of the pregnancy to encourage movement and towards a naturally induced labour. It is very effective during the labour too to speed up contractions. Acupressure can be applied during the labour.

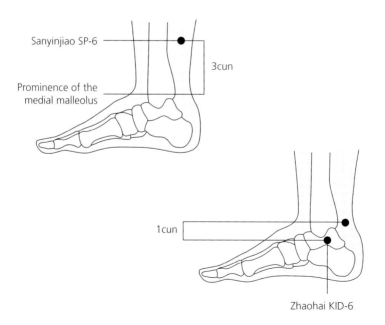

Ren-4 Guan Yuan (Gate of Origin)

Ren-4 Guan Yuan is another important point. In other traditions like yoga you may have heard this referred to as the 'hara'. This point has many actions, it benefits the Uterus directly and assists conception.

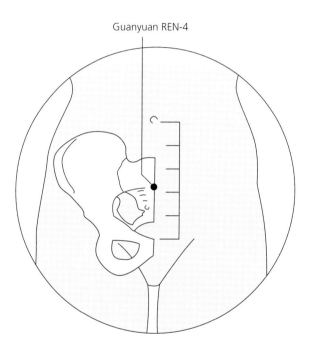

Guanyuan REN-4

St-36 Zu San Li (Leg Three Miles)

This is the single most important point to stimulate the Stomach and Spleen in generating Qi and Blood. It tonifies the Qi of the whole body.

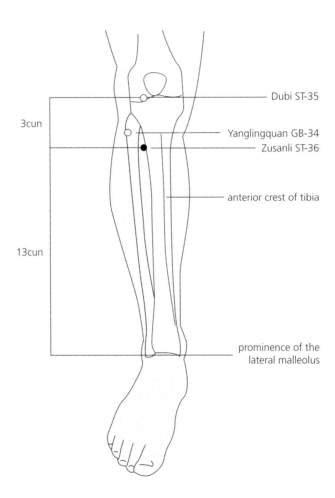

Liv-3 Tai Chong (Great Rushing)

This is an effective point to free up any tension in the body. Any indications of frustration or anger will be relieved by needling this point. It also helps to free the Blood.

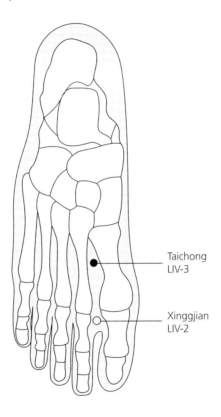

Taichong
LIV-3

Xinggjian
LIV-2

Remember this is only a small selection of acupuncture points to give you a flavour of acupuncture. Your acupuncturist will make a diagnosis based on what they see that day. A TCM (Traditional Chinese Medicine) Acupuncturist will look at your tongue and also take your pulse. They will select the points that seem relevant to them for you. They are like the artist standing at the easel, choosing the colours that are best for you. Often bringing more colour, lightness and sense of ease to your world!

About Amanda Thomas

Amanda Thomas has been practising acupuncture since 2005 and specialises in gynaecological issues and fertility/infertility using Chinese herbs. She also treats babies and children with a gentle Japanese technique called Shonishin. She is passionate about wellbeing and sharing an understanding around how the mind works through the work of Sydney Banks.

When she isn't doing this, she is an artist, enjoys yoga, walking and travelling. She is a Mum to a beautiful spirit and is hopeful that enough people will wake up to save our wonderful planet for future generations.

"Out beyond ideas of wrongdoing and right doings, there is a field.

I'll meet you there.

When the soul lies down in that grass,

the world is too full to talk about.

Ideas, language, even the phrase 'each other' doesn't make any sense."

Rumi

Always meet you there! Amanda is available for heart felt conversations online as well as acupuncture in person.

www.hummingbirdacupuncture.co.uk

Acknowledgements

Thank you to all the Gurus who submitted chapters for this book

Thanks to Pops (Bob Sheehan) for the myriad of tasks that he does to enable me to focus on my work – making dinner, taking the orders to the post office to name a few.

Thanks too to my sister Lu (Laura Sheehan) who is my biggest cheerleader, financial backer and surprise pressie giver.

Thanks to my brother Greg who kept Pops busy during Covid-19 lockdown and dragged me out for walks when staring at a screen got too much, and when lockdown got too much for him, he took over my book orders, packaging, posting, and even cleared out the garage ready for my new delivery of books.

Thanks to Nicki Averill who works her magic on my raw documents and turns them into a thing of beauty.

Thanks to Alison McCalpin PR who makes sure that you hear about the books.

Thanks to Kerry Richards who helped a guru finesse their work.

Thanks to Doreen Chin Ling (https://www.bellessence.co.uk/) who proofreads like a dream.

Thanks to all my students – past, present and future – without you, there would be no books.

Thank you to Dawn Emmerson, my foot model, who suffers willingly for my art!

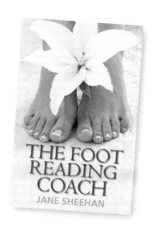
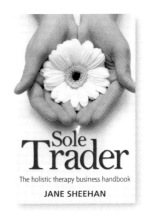

Lisons nos pieds!

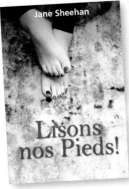

Tous que vous voulez savoir au sujet de la lecture des pieds. Qu'est ce que vos pieds vous dites de vos émotions et personnalité?

Voici le premier livre de la série écrite par Jane pour vous apprendre à « lire les pieds ».

Découvrez si vous êtes une princesse ou un cheval de trait.

Que disent vos verrues sur vous?

Pourquoi ne parvenez-vous pas à vous débarrasser de votre pied d'athlète?

Pour quelles raisons la pantoufle de vair de Cendrillon ne pouvait-elle pas lui aller?

Prix spécial disponible sur ce site uniquement:
£ 14 + frais de port

www.lecturedespieds.fr
ISBN 978-0-9571071-1-3

Also available in Italian language: Leggiamoci I Piedi
www.letturadeipiedi.it
ISBN 978-1-8381134-1-4

Foot Reading – The Portable Guide

These hand-held reference cards are exclusive to our website. After Jane Sheehan produced her foot reading poster, she was often asked whether a hand-held version was available. As a result she produced this portable guide.

It acts as an aide-memoire to her first book "Let's Read Our Feet!" and the information is laid out in the order you would need it when conducting a foot reading.

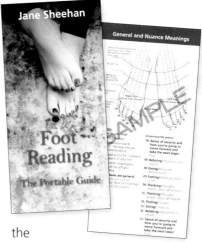

The cards consist of eighteen 210mm x 100mm laminated cards held together by a metal post and printed only on one side so that you can swivel them open to quickly find the information that you need. As the cards are laminated they're easy to wipe clean – a bonus when you're working with feet!

£12 plus postage and packaging
Available exclusively from www.footreading.com

Also available in French language:
Lisons nos pieds – le guide portable
ISBN 978-0-9571071-3-7
www.lecturedespieds.fr

The Foot Reading Poster

This is an A3 sized glossy poster detailing different aspects of foot reading and including the emotional map of the dorsal and plantar aspects of the foot. It's clear, concise and beautifully illustrated. It's a good companion to the book "Let's Read our Feet!"

Available from www.footreading.com
ISBN 978-0-9550593-5-3
£12.00 + post and packing

Also available in French language:
L'affiche de la lecture des pieds
ISBN 978-0-95710711-3-3
www.lecturedespieds.fr

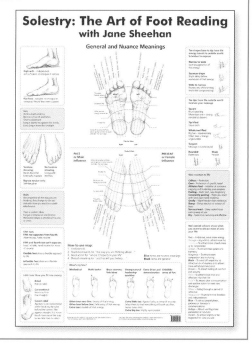

The Gurus' Guide to Reflexology Series:

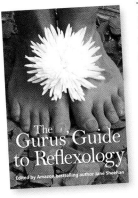

These books are designed to introduce the reflexologist to the many different forms of reflexology showing the progression of the therapy. Each book is divided into two sections. The first section is the collection of chapters from the "gurus" writing about their specialisms and the second section includes information that will support the reflexologist and their client.

Book 1: 17 Gurus showing the many forms of reflexology
ISBN 978 0-9571071-5-1
Book 2: themed on the topic of hormones. 13 Gurus share their knowledge to aid puberty, infertility, fertility, pregnancy, and menopause ISBN 978 0-9571071-6-8
Book 3: theme on the topic of cancer.
ISBN 978-0-9571071-7-5

For more information see www.footreading.com

Also available in French Language
Le guide des gourous pour la réflexologie, Livre 1
ISBN 978-1-8381134-0-7
www.lecturedespieds.fr

Animal Reflexology Poster

This A3 sized laminated poster shows the Animal Reflexology points on both the front and hind "feet" and is a beautiful companion to the chapter on Animal Reflexology by Yvette Eastman in The Gurus' Guide to Reflexology Book 1. The points shown are suitable for cats, dogs and horses.

ISBN 3978-0-9571071-8-2
Cost is £12 plus P&P
See www.footreading.com

Also available in French language
Tableau << Main>> et << Pied >> de l'Animal
ISBN 978-0-9571071-9-9
www.lecturedespieds.fr

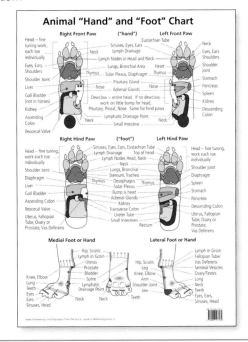

Motivation Cards
(similar to former Inspiration cards)

Motivation Cards (like Inspiration Cards) with photos on one side and quotations on the other.

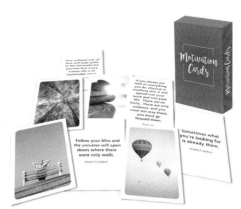

In Jane's books she talks about using "Inspiration Cards" at the end of her foot readings. Those cards are no longer available.

So Jane decided to make her own version because they are, in her words "a valuable part of my foot reading tool kit".

They are designed to be used in several ways:

1 Projection
2 For Creative Writing
3 Goal setting
4 Daily meditation
5 Up to you: Maybe you can think of other ways to use the cards too.

£12.50 plus postage and packaging
ISBN-13-978-0-957107

Available from www.footreading.com

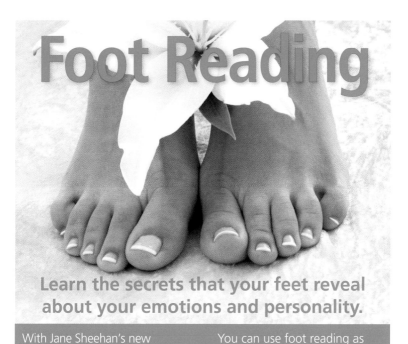

Foot Reading

Learn the secrets that your feet reveal about your emotions and personality.

With Jane Sheehan's new **e-learning seminar**, now you can learn to read feet in your own time at your own pace and even in your pyjamas if you want to!

You can use foot reading as
■ a therapy in its own right
■ to add to an existing therapy
■ or just to amaze your friends

See www.footreading.com/elearning.htm for details

See Jane Live

List of workshops at www.footreading.com
If you have a group of 10 or more and would like to organise one of Jane's workshops, ring

07739 802175 or email jane@footreading.com